Purge
rehab diaries

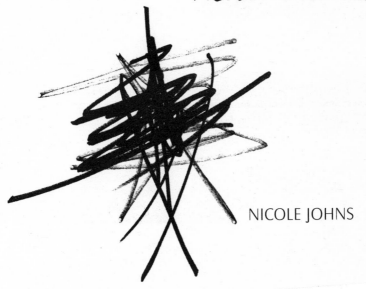

NICOLE JOHNS

D0122036

SEAL PRESS

Purge
REHAB DIARIES

Copyright © 2009 by Nicole Johns

Published by
Seal Press
A Member of Perseus Books Group
1700 Fourth Street
Berkeley, California

Library of Congress Cataloging-in-Publication Data

Johns, Nicole.
  Purge : rehab diaries / Nicole Johns.
    p. cm.
  ISBN-13: 978-1-58005-274-0
  ISBN-10: 1-58005-274-6
  1. Johns, Nicole—Health. 2. Eating disorders—Patients—United States—Biography. 3. Eating disorders—Patients—Services for—United States. I. Title.
  RC552.E18J64 2009
  362.196'85260092—dc22
  [B]
                              2008041319

Cover and interior design by Domini Dragoone
Printed in the United States of America by Maple-Vail
Distributed by Publishers Group West

The information contained in this book is for general interest only. The author is not a physician, and no information found here should be used for medical purposes—diagnostically, therapeutically, or as a substitute for the advice provided by your own medical professional. In order to respect the privacy of individuals mentioned in this book, the author has changed their names.

DEDICATION

For those who haven't found their way out yet;
and for those of us who have,
and will always remember.

Contents

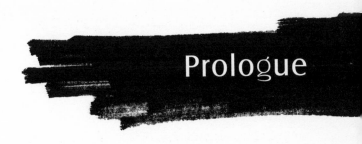

Prologue

We are, I am, you are
by cowardice or courage
the one who find our way
back to this scene . . .

—FROM "DIVING INTO THE WRECK,"

BY ADRIENNE RICH

have used adrienne rich's poem

I have used Adrienne Rich's poem "Diving into the Wreck" as a metaphor to describe the process of writing this book, as well as my recovery from an eating disorder. I have had to dive into the wreck of my journals, my medical and psychiatric records, the minds of those who accompanied me during my three months of treatment, and my own mind in order to find my way back to the scene and accurately record my experience. I chose to write about the three months I spent in residential treatment for Eating Disorder Not Otherwise Specified (EDNOS) because there is a dearth of well-written, timely, and accurate literature about eating disorder treatment.

Numerous psychological studies have been published regarding the success rates of various methods of treating eating disorders. While such studies are integral to healthcare professionals' understanding of how to better treat eating-disordered individuals, they do not tell the story of the individual who struggles with an eating disorder, or her treatment experience.[1] Although a recent explosion of self-help books addresses the topic of eating disorders, these books often offer dubious advice and are poorly written.

Another genre of eating disorder books exists: a cross between the traditional self-help book and the memoir. In these books, the narrator is "saved" by a treatment provider or God, or a combination of both. These books give the reader the impression that an eating disorder is just a diet gone wrong, and that it can be cured if the individual finds the right support group, the right religion, or the right therapist.

Unfortunately, it is not that simple. Eating disorders are complex pathologies—they do not stem from a single source, they have no simple resolution, and they are seldom cured. Treatment can help an individual lessen her symptoms (restricting, purging, and so on) and obtain a better quality of life. However, treatment does not cure an eating disorder. What the general public does not realize is that the eating-disordered individual struggles and needs continued support after leaving treatment, and that, to some extent, she will struggle with eating disorder urges after treatment, even if she doesn't act on them. The happily ever after ending of many of the eating disorder books on the market today is a myth.

One of my main goals in writing this book is to reveal that despite having spent three months in treatment, I am not cured, and neither are the majority of patients. I wanted to write an honest, detailed narrative about my experience in treatment and the effect it had on my life. I wanted to show the reader that there is no happily ever after, but that there is hope. Most of the current eating disorder literature glosses over the ugly parts of living with and attempting to recover from an eating disorder. I chose specifically to describe what it is like to purge, what it is like to abuse diet pills and starve myself. The readers deserve to know the truth, rather than have it sugar-coated. For this reason, I also included a number of primary documents from my stint in treatment. Along with aiding the structure of my book, these documents detail my treatment experience and offer the reader a clearer idea of the treatment process.

Most of the literature about eating disorders written by treatment providers and individuals who have battled an eating disorder creates the unrealistic expectation that the reader's eating disorder will be cured after one round of treatment, after a few therapy sessions, or after the eating-disordered individual reaches a healthy weight or stops purging. The reality of eating disorder treatment is that the relapse rate is astronomical. According to the Cleveland Clinic, up to 50 percent of bulimics relapse six months after treatment, and the relapse rate for anorexia is even higher.[2]

We as readers are living in the age of the memoir. Memoirs, especially those dealing with subjects previously deemed taboo by society, are selling well. Eating disorders have not gone undocumented in this era.

The preeminent eating disorder memoir is *Wasted*, by Marya Hornbacher. As a senior in college, I checked out *Wasted* from the library and read the book in one day, as I was riveted by Hornbacher's description of her battle(s) with anorexia and bulimia. At the time, I was in the throes of purging anorexia—my goal was to eat less than seven hundred calories a day; I purged if I exceeded my self-imposed limit, in an effort to lose weight and gain control over something in my life: my body.

It is worth noting that *Wasted* has a cult following of eating-disordered individuals. While I was in treatment, several women attempted to smuggle *Wasted* into the treatment facility, but the staff confiscated their dog-eared copies of the book. These women considered *Wasted* their eating disorder bible; they gleaned tips from it and used it to trigger their own eating disorder behaviors.

The cover of *Wasted* was what first caught my attention. The paperback edition of the book showcases a thin Hornbacher on its front cover. To non-eating-disordered women, this visual of the author and what she has done to her body may serve as a warning. But all I saw was that she was thin.

As a reader, I searched for firsthand accounts of what life in a treatment center is like, and was left unsatisfied. As I progressed through treatment, I learned that I was not the only one without a clear idea of what eating disorder treatment entails. Well-meaning friends thought it was like summer camp, while others thought

I'd be spending time on lockdown with psychotic individuals. The reality of the treatment experience (or at least my treatment experience) was quite different from what most people imagine. My hope is that this book dispels the myths about eating disorder treatment that are circulating.

Another myth I hope to dispel is that anyone who is not emaciated cannot have an eating disorder. At 137 pounds, in the midst of consuming diet-pill cocktails, starving, and purging, I was hospitalized for fainting, a concussion, electrolyte imbalances, and three different kinds of heart-rhythm irregularities. My eating disorder behavior had wreaked havoc on my body. Not until after treatment did I learn the sum total of the damage I had done, but for a long time I refused to believe I had a problem because I was not underweight.

In treatment, I met overweight and normal-weight bulimics with an array of medical problems—including heart irregularities, eroded esophageal tracts, bowel problems, osteopenia, and osteoporosis—at the age of twenty. A person does not have to be underweight to suffer the medical consequences (not to mention the emotional pain) of an eating disorder. An eating-disordered individual should not have to weigh fifty-two pounds to be taken seriously.

In conclusion, I wrote this book to inform the public, counteract the myths surrounding eating disorders and treatment, and provide eating-disordered individuals with hope.

1. While most eating disorder patients are female, it should be noted that increasing numbers of males are seeking treatment for eating disorders.
2. http://www.clevelandclinicmeded.com

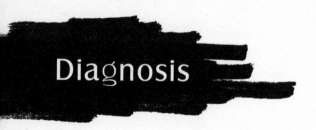

Diagnosis

Eating Disorder Not Otherwise Specified
(EDNOS),
characterized by restricting and purging.

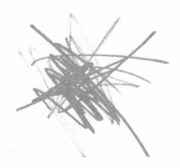

(2001—2004)

Selected Journal Entries

made myself sick and it felt really
ood

12/10/01: I made myself sick and it felt really good. I liked it.
I'm one sick fuck.

12/21/01: 143 lbs. I feel disgusting. I look disgusting.
I need to lose at least 10 lbs.

6/13/02: 139 lbs. Bulimia is back. I've started taking
diet pills with ephedra.

6/29/02: I threw up my birthday dinner.

7/3/02: I threw up every day last week.

7/7/02: Threw up uncooked brownie mix. That was sick.

9/24/02: I've developed heart problems from bulimia and diet pills.

10/11/02: 144 lbs. Reading Marya Hornbacher's *Wasted*.

10/19/02: Dizziness and chest pain when I purged.

10/27/02: I feel myself slowly slipping into anorexia. I'm in the
interim. No pills, less purging. A gradual changeover.
I'm remembering my summer of compulsive running. I'm
remembering my blood pressure bottoming out at boarding school because I wasn't eating. Exhaustion. Dizziness.
Running around jacketless in winter so I would burn more
calories. My body has lost its integrity. Binged at Perkins,
and then threw it all up.

1/11/03: 135 lbs. Therapist claims I'm emaciated. Wants me to
watch a Lifetime movie.

2/28/03: 130 lbs. I'm focused on my plunge into bulimia and
anorexia. It's been a hellish past few months in that respect.
My hair is falling out, my nails are a mess, I'm dizzy and
on the verge of passing out a lot. I look like shit, except I'm

thinner, and everyone notices and the compliments keep rolling in the more I drop. I need the muscle spasms and irregular heartbeat to stop.

4/17/03: 141 lbs. I have wasted a year of my life. The year that held so much promise in the beginning. All the time I spent counting calories and purging has been a waste. I haven't purged in a month. Not worrying about food gives me so much time. I can eat dinner with my friends. Eating disorders are a subtle suicide, and I am choosing to live.

4/29/03: I slipped. I binged and purged.

9/13/03: Started taking diet pills again. Feel so gross. Some things never change.

9/21/03: 150 lbs. That's three-quarters of the way to 200. Fatness. I'm going to take diet pills and stay under 1,000 calories a day.

1/31/04: 138 lbs. The only time I'm hungry is when I wake up in the morning. Then I eat, take a Metabolife, and have energy, but not hunger. I know this is completely ridiculous, but if I can just get down to 100 lbs., then I can start over and do everything right. I see this as getting to the essentials, the basics. Looking in the mirror today, I noticed I looked thinner. It was nice. At 138, I don't look too bad, and at 128, I'd look even better. It's been so easy lately with these pills, having three classes and one section to teach. Starving=happy, binge/purge=unhappy. I'm finally starting to figure it out.

2/4/04: I am in too deep now. Half the time I feel like I don't have anything the matter with me because it's not physically evident. Then I feel guilty about eating. I just don't know. I'm ashamed because I'm too old for this. I am scared that I'm never going to get better. Worse, I'm scared I'll stay in the exact same place. . . . Mirrors lie. There are fat mirrors and skinny mirrors; which ones are right? Now I know I'm happier, because not eating=control. And I hide the disorders so well. I'm a pro. No one needs to know. My guilty secret. It's my Incredible Shrinking Woman act. I want to shrink into oblivion. Get to the bare bones, the essentials. I throw up my emotions. My grief, my secrets. I starve away into nothingness, flatness.

2/11/04: I feel like I'm going to pass out. I'm eating two candy bars. I feel like I'm losing my mind. This is madness. Since I've eaten these candy bars, I'm only allowed salad tonight. I have my life all together, except for this. Maybe I should purge these candy bars. Now I want a muffin. I just want to go to bed, but I can't sleep anymore.

3/28/04: Sometimes I hate what I've reduced my life to.

4/4/04: I feel like I'm dying.

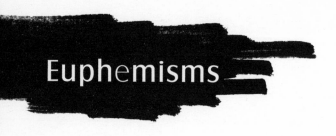

Euphemisms

ing yourself sick, purging,
ing, scarf and barf,
induced vomiting,
ing in bulimic symptoms,
ing, Making yourself sick, purging, yakking, scarf and barf, self-
pulsi induced vomiting, engaging in bulimic symptoms. Starving, restrict-
in an ing, fasting, compulsive exercising, engaging in anorexic symptoms.
None of these terms adequately describe the frenzy of an eating
disorder. An eating disorder, to most people, is anorexia or bulimia.
But, there is an island between anorexia and bulimia, a no-man's-
land that borrows from both diagnoses. This island is Eating Disorder Not Otherwise Specified (EDNOS).[1]

An eating disorder is driving to a gas station in the midst of
a blizzard and writing a bad check to buy dozens of stale doughnuts because they are being sold at the day-old discount price and

you are ravenous because you have been starving yourself, again. Your car gets stuck in the middle of an intersection, your tires churn up wet snow, you're going nowhere as you cram doughnuts into your mouth, sugar circling your lips and chin, granules of sticky sugar on the steering wheel, and you don't care that there is oncoming traffic, the light is about to change, and the tires are spinning. All you care about is making it back to the apartment before your roommate gets off work, in time to stick the index finger of your right hand down your inflamed throat so that doughnut pieces will heave their way up your esophagus and plummet into the toilet bowl.

Back at the apartment, your right hand is slick with saliva, mucus, and chunks of wet doughnut. Your eyes water and tears roll down your face and land in the toilet bowl, mixing with the doughnut remains. There is a splash-back effect as the doughnut pieces hit the water. Toilet water splashes your face but you don't care, because all you can think of are calories, fat grams, *did I get it all out?* Then you strip down, running your hands over the contour of your hips; you search for rib bones and shoulder blades, and you grab the loose skin of your abdomen in disgust.

An eating disorder is bingeing on a salad with fat-free dressing in the student union, running up three flights of stairs to a seldom-used bathroom, and pausing to look in the mirror before going into a stall. Eyes are ringed with circles, lips are chapped, there's a scar on your right knuckle from where your teeth scrape when you shove your fingers down your throat. You are pale. You retch away, the acidic salad dressing burning your throat and mouth; wilted brown lettuce coated with a sheen of bile glides back up your blistered throat.

Ten minutes before seminar starts, you race to Starbucks, buy a large black coffee, dump three Equals into it, and walk to class, wondering, *When is my body going to give out?* It's negative ten degrees outside, goddamn Minnesota, but you are oblivious, coat unbuttoned, scarf trailing off your shoulder. The hand holding your coffee shakes. In the bathroom of the English building you gulp down two Dexatrims with your coffee, sitting through seminar in a glazed stupor, anxious and paranoid, voice wavering, neck and face turning a splotchy red if you attempt to contribute to the class discussion.

The scale is waiting when you come home from school. The scale is always waiting. You tentatively step on, and red neon numbers blink back at you. Down three pounds. Hands shaking, eyes red, you're breathing rapidly and your heart is on overdrive, thumping against the confines of your rib cage.

You wake up in the night, almost every night, terrified that you've gained weight. At three o'clock on a frigid winter morning, you leave the nest of your blanketed bed and slide out of flannel pajamas. Shivering, you pull the scale out from its hiding place under your bed and step on. You haven't gained ten pounds in your sleep. You go back to bed.

1. *The Diagnostic and Statistical Manual of Mental Disorders, Fourth Edition,* published in 2000, includes the following diagnostic criteria for EDNOS:

All of the criteria for anorexia nervosa are met, except the individual has regular menses.

All of the criteria for anorexia nervosa are met, except that despite substantial weight loss, the individual's current weight is in the normal range.

All of the criteria for bulimia nervosa are met, except binges occur at a frequency of less than twice a week or for a duration of less than three months.

An individual of normal body weight who regularly engages in inappropriate compensatory behavior after eating small amounts of food (e.g., self-induced vomiting after consuming two cookies).

An individual who repeatedly chews and spits out, and does not swallow, large amounts of food.

Binge eating disorder; recurrent episodes of binge eating in the absence of the regular use of inappropriate compensatory behaviors characteristic of bulimia nervosa.

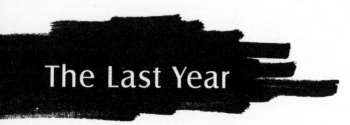

The Last Year

(OF YOUR LOVE AFFAIR WITH EDNOS)

You are twenty-two and have never lived in a big city or the Midwest. You come to Minnesota armed with your BA in English and gender studies from Penn State Erie, and a history of winning scholarships and awards. You think you've left the past behind, hidden in the mountains of rural Pennsylvania. You couldn't be more wrong.

You build an impressive facade, claiming that you aren't homesick, that you are happy and love Minnesota. These are all blatant, flagrant lies.

There are times when you can almost love Minnesota for its vast flatness, its strange breed of liberalism, and the immense blueness of its sky. But you can't get past the crackheads on the corner of Franklin and Clinton Avenues; you can't get past the fact that it is never quiet and never dark in this strange, flat land where people butcher their vowels when they speak.

You turn awkward and quiet, again.

Buy a scale at Target. See the numbers and go into shock. Buy diet pills. Screw the heart problems—you'll get thin or die trying.

The Incredible Shrinking Woman act begins, again.

Restrict, tabulate, and calculate calories. Pop ephedra-laced diet pills like candy. Any time you go over your self-imposed caloric limit, purge. At first the limit is one thousand calories, then eight hundred, then six hundred, then five hundred. Begin purging constantly. You think you've hit bottom, but you haven't.

Start running by the Mississippi River because it's the closest thing you have to Lake Erie. Run until you're spent. Then it starts snowing and you have to stop running.

At 8:00 AM, catch the number 20 bus and go to school. The Somali women on Cedar Avenue wrap themselves in scarves and flowing fabrics. You are almost jealous. You wish you could hide your body in folds of flowing fabric.

The University of Minnesota is loud and sprawling, with traffic and swarms of people. Scurry to Lind Hall; the English department is your refuge. Type away in the graduate-student computer lab. Story after story, lesson plan after lesson plan, poem after poem.

Make it a goal to not eat at school. And don't. Instead, wash down diet pills with large coffees diluted with five Equals. You shake a lot, your pupils are always dilated, and dark circles ring your eyes. Your body is exhausted but your mind is on overdrive.

You pull off this plunge because everyone is unaware. It takes a while for the questions and confrontations to start.

Meanwhile, you are losing—yourself, your mind, and, most important, weight. You have condensed your life down to two things: weight loss and school.

The baristas at Caribou Coffee on Washington Avenue know you by name because you spend your weekends there, grading papers and writing in your journal while consuming strong coffee. If you're not at Caribou, you are downtown on Nicollet Mall, wandering through the streets, staring up at skyscrapers, reminding yourself that you live in a city and never have to go back to your isolated hometown in Pennsylvania.

But you do go back. In November you break down and buy a $300 plane ticket you can't afford, to Erie, Pennsylvania, where you went to college. You have a fabulous time there. It hits you how much you miss Erie. You take a guy home from the bar to make Carla jealous. Carla is in love with you and you are in love with Carla, although neither of you will ever act on it because she is forty and married. Your ploy works. Carla is jealous. You and Carla never really speak again.

Carla's letters were the only things that got you through some days and now, suddenly, they are gone.

It grows bitterly cold in Minneapolis. At negative thirty-five degree windchill, the tears on your eyelashes freeze. You feel even fatter because you have to wear long underwear and so many layers.

One of your roommates has friends coming in from Wisconsin for Thanksgiving. You think it will be a lonely holiday for you, but you fall in love the day before.

Her name is Diana and she's a tall, redheaded Minnesotan. She persuades you to go dancing at Lucy's Bar, but you don't so much dance as make out. She is five-foot-nine, and at five-foot-five, you have to stand on tiptoe to reach her lips.

Her scent is lavender. You are enamored. Your friends drive both of you back to your house at 2:00 AM; it's you and Diana in the back seat, kissing, while your friend drives through the deserted streets of St. Paul, where the hard, granular snow glistens in the light of the streetlamps.

The sun rises before the two of you fall asleep, a mess of tangled limbs in your tangled sheets.

At first, Diana is a weekend event. Then she calls you every night and you grow overwhelmed; she is too close. You talk about this and she backs off.

You always have a bottle of wine waiting for Diana, as well as fresh sheets. It's all very romantic. Your Minnesota friends like Diana. You meet her parents. But you don't tell her your secrets.

Diana's skin is a winter white, paler than your own skin. The two of you lie on navy blue sheets; her head rests on your chest while you twist strands of her auburn hair around your index finger. It's snowing again, and you listen to the wind scour the plains.

"Your heart is beating out of rhythm," she says.

"I know."

"Why does it do that?"

Shift her off your chest and kiss her.

Then, on a frigid January morning, she breaks up with you. Now she's the one who feels stifled. You binge and purge the day away at McDonald's. Then you start drinking. You are hungover and depressed from purging and drinking.

People start noticing that you aren't all right. You keep losing weight and you look like hell. One of your friends in the English department is the first to confront you in the grocery store Rainbow Foods on East Lake Street. She stares you down in the canned-goods aisle and asks whether you are bulimic, anorexic, or a little bit of both. You think for a moment and say a little bit of both. She glances in your cart and shakes her head. Your cart contains a tub of fat-free plain yogurt, a bag of salad, cans of vegetables, a bunch of bananas, and a half-gallon of skim milk.

You don't realize how out of control you are, even after you fall down a flight of stairs in the English department. Much to your relief, no one sees you fall.

Spring semester, you take Memory and Memoir and Poetry of Social Change classes. You love both of these classes and actually start talking in them. You have found your voice again. You enjoy the challenge of reading Proust and Nabokov, and you love working at St. Stephen's Men's Shelter through Poetry of Social Change. It makes you feel like you have some self-worth. Sometimes it makes you feel incredibly guilty as you walk through the ghetto, dressed in a warm coat and waterproof shoes, in subzero weather. The inhabitants of the ghetto have none of this.

One impenetrable Midwestern night, you are desperate because you are trapped in your life. There is no way out, so you binge on and purge an entire tube of Pillsbury rolls (half-cooked— you are too impatient to wait for them to bake), an entire box of chocolate Malt-O-Meal, a pint of Godiva ice cream, and a mug of chai tea. Though you know that constant purging and starving leads to dehydration, you don't rehydrate when you're done.

In bed, you can't sleep. Your heart is skittering erratically. You wonder if you're dying. Maybe you won't wake up in the morning. Maybe that wouldn't be so bad.

You do wake up the next morning, and you have a bulimic hangover because you are so dehydrated and malnourished. The world spins, your head aches, your heart throbs hard in your chest, and you almost pass out in the shower. You think about canceling the class you teach, but don't.

After your shower, you dress, then reach to get your cell phone off the table in your room. You lose your balance and fall to the floor, smacking your head on the corner of the table. Instantly, you vomit. You remember this is a sign of a concussion, so you call a cab to take you to the health center.

By the time the cab arrives, you've grabbed your insurance card, jacket, cell phone, and keys. You sit on the curb, head in your hands, sobbing.

At the student health center they take one look at you and start an IV. They think you have the flu and you let them believe this. They are concerned—you're dehydrated, your electrolytes are a mess, and your already low blood pressure plummets when you stand up. They think you have a concussion and they send you to the ER.

You are admitted to the cardiology unit because you are having premature atrial contractions, premature ventricular contractions, and bradycardia. All of these heart irregularities are direct results of your eating disorder. You call home to Pennsylvania because you think it's the right thing to do. You are scared. The cardiologist tells you this is all a result of purging, starving, and diet pills. You tell your parents it's just stress; there is no need to worry them with the truth.

The doctors release you from the hospital the next day, and it is apparent that you have a concussion. Typing is an ordeal, as are most cognitive functions. All you want to do is sleep.

You realize you are going through the motions of life. You are running literally on black coffee and diet pills. Everyone is concerned about your hospitalization. Later, you find out no one bought your story about having the flu.

Your poetry professor drives you home every Tuesday night after seminar. She pulls up in front of your house and peers at you. She wants to know what is really going on. You hop out of the car and thank her for her concern, but you are just fine.

At this point, you wonder if you've lost your mind. All you

think about is food and school. You think things can't get any worse, but they do.

It's seven o'clock on a Sunday morning, the last day in February. You answer your cell phone and your father tells you your uncle has been killed in a car wreck. His ancient Blazer slid on the winter-slick gravel roads of home, flipped, and rolled into a dark ravine. You fly home. You are numb; you don't believe this is really happening. You go to his gravesite in an icy March rain and say goodbye. You finally cry there.

You stay home for a week after your uncle dies. You don't want to fly back to Minnesota, but the hills of Pennsylvania are suffocating, so you go back.

You start attending eating disorder group therapy at the student health center the next week, but quit shortly after you start. Someone always cried during group therapy, which made you grip the arms of your chair, not sure how to react. Group was a strange place where the unofficial motto was "I'm okay, you're okay, and we're all just okay." This was supposed to help, to show that you were not alone. Group was part of your mental-health maintenance. Going every week, setting goals, and acknowledging setbacks were supposed to help you get better.

In group, you talked about food and feelings; you lay stretched out on the floor and tried to imagine a time when you were happy with your body. Your mind drifted to the green hills of home and the drought-dry tall grass that lines the back field by the edge of the cliff. You remember searching for sun-ripened raspberries in the abandoned chicken coop, the searing midday sun on your bare shoulders. You were eight and sturdy. Your body was yours, no one had trespassed upon it, and you valued the steady beat of your heart.

You drifted back into the reality of the urban landscape outside the group therapy room, to the sound of rush-hour traffic hurtling down the street. The women talked about their memories of a time before the vigilance of eating disorders, but your mind fixated on the memory of your eight-year-old self.

Your therapist urges you to enter a treatment program. You tell yourself you are just fine.

Meanwhile, because you are so miserable, you are praying for a gastric rupture or the chance to die in your sleep. Your therapist claims you are passively suicidal, and you tell her an eating disorder is a slow, painful suicide. An eating disorder is an abusive lover you keep crawling back to. You wonder if you can break the cycle. You call your insurance provider, BlueCross BlueShield of Minnesota, and ask if they cover residential eating disorder treatment (a woman from group therapy has recommended residential treatment over treatment in the local hospital). They do. You qualify. You don't even have to pay a copayment, because the powers that be have deemed treatment medically necessary. And so you order your train ticket, $76 from Minneapolis to Milwaukee, and on May 24 you decide to give life a try, again.

The End Is the Beginning

I spend my last night of freedom in the 400 Bar in Minneapolis,
swaying to an unknown band, a plastic cup of lukewarm Sam
Adams in one hand, a cigarette I bummed off someone in the other.
In three months, the jeans I'm wearing, my favorite pair of size 9
jeans that fit just right, won't fit me. This is the last beer I will drink
for over three months. I haven't left for treatment yet, but somehow
I sense this is the end of something; this last night at the bar has a
sense of finality to it.

Someone spills beer on my shirt and I want to ask the
bartender on a date, but he's got a girlfriend and I'm leaving for
treatment in Wisconsin tomorrow. Back at my house, I pack

halfheartedly. My roommates are out celebrating the end of the semester, so I am alone. I swallow some Dexatrims that I wash down with a Diet Coke chaser because I know at this time tomorrow, I won't be allowed to have either. Dexatrims and Diet Coke are considered contraband at the Eating Disorders Center. I imagine friendly nurses with squeaky white shoes catching me with the Dexatrims I'm planning on sneaking in. In my imagination, the nurses let me keep the pills because they see that I need them. They see that I am fat.

Around 2:00 AM, I make an entire box of chocolate Malt-O-Meal with skim milk and a gluttonous amount of white sugar. I eat all of this viscous, syrupy-sweet concoction and then frantically search the cupboards for something to binge on, but there is nothing to eat. I sprint to my room in search of my scale, forgetting that a friend confiscated it this morning. I am paranoid that I have gained weight from the beer and the Malt-O-Meal and the brunch I had with friends earlier in the day. I chug Diet Coke and head to the bathroom and retch until there is nothing left in my stomach.

I lie awake in bed, jittery with caffeine and insomnia. My heart races and thumps in an unsteady beat. I should care, but I don't. Part of me wishes for cardiac arrest because I don't know how I'm going to let go of this.

My alarm goes off at 5:30 AM, and I wait for the cab to pick me up and take me to the Amtrak station. As the train lurches out of St. Paul, I mutter, "Goodbye, Minnesota" because I don't think I'm coming back. I don't eat all day, and wash diet pills down with

Diet Coke at regular intervals as the train speeds south and east. I'm lulled by the soothing rocking motion and fall into a stupor, staring at the lush greenness of late spring in the Midwest. I can't read or write; all I can do is watch Minnesota fade into Wisconsin.

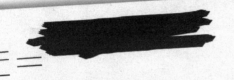

INPATIENT AUTHORIZATION

Inpatient admission has been authorized for:
Patient: JOHNS, NICOLE J
Identification #:
Member #: 0000
Relation to subscriber: SUBSCRIBER
Sex: FEMALE   Date of birth: 06-29-81

NICOLE   J JOHNS

This admission has been authorized for:
Hospital:
Date of admission: 05-24-04

The day of admission has been authorized beginning   05-24-04 . This notification fulfills the preadmis
notification requirement in the subscriber contract.

TO THE PATIENT:

Please note the following conditions which apply to this authorization:

- Your contract provides benefits for an inpatient stay as long as the level of care being provided i
  medically necessary. This means the patient's condition must require an acute inpatient level of care
- We will be contacting the admitting/treating physician and/or facility for updates or requesting and
  reviewing medical records. It is important that we receive updates and/or medical records when rec
- Expenses related to all days found not to require the acute inpatient level may be your responsibili
- If you have questions regarding your contract benefits, please contact your Customer Service Depar
  _____ OR _____ .

TO THE TREATING PROVIDER/FACILITY:

Please note the following conditions which apply to this authorization:

- The subscriber's contract provides benefits for an inpatient stay as long as the level of care bei
  provided is medically necessary. This means the patient's condition must require an acute inpatient
  care.
- We will be contacting you for updates or requesting and reviewing medical records. It is importa
  receive the updates and/or medical records when requested.
- If you have questions regarding the subscribers contract benefits, please contact the Provider Se

Please note the following conditions which ...

- Your contract provides benefits for an inpatient stay as long as the ... medically necessary. This means the patient's condition must require an acute inpa... ...
- We will be contacting the admitting/treating physician and/or facility for updates or requesting ... reviewing medical records. It is important that we receive updates and/or medical records when requested.
- Expenses related to all days found not to require the acute inpatient level may be your responsibility.
- If you have questions regarding your contract benefits, please contact your Customer Service Department at ▬▬▬▬ OR ▬▬▬▬.

TO THE TREATING PROVIDER/FACILITY:

Please note the following conditions which apply to this authorization:

- The subscriber's contract provides benefits for an inpatient stay as long as the level of care being provided is medically necessary. This means the patient's condition must require an acute inpatient level of care.
- We will be contacting you for updates or requesting and reviewing medical records. It is important that we receive the updates and/or medical records when requested.
- If you have questions regarding the subscribers contract benefits, please contact the Provider Service Department at ▬▬▬▬ OR ▬▬▬▬.

Utilization Management has approved the service requested as medically necessary, however this does not guarantee payment of the claim. Final payment of benefits is based on the contract that is in force on the day services are received and whether premiums have been paid, lifetime or benefits maximums have been exceeded, the condition treated is not a pre—existing condition, the service authorized is the service billed and the provider is eligible for reimbursement. Failure to use a Participating Provider may result in additio... financial liability.

For specific subscriber/patient benefit information, you must call the customer service or provider service numbers listed on the back of the membership identification card.

If you have any questions regarding this notification process, please contact Medical Services Administr...
▬▬▬▬ or ▬▬▬▬

Welcome

The staff of the Eating Disorder Center at ▬▬▬▬▬▬▬ welcomes you. We would like to assist you during this difficult time by identifying your strengths and evaluating those areas causing you concern.

We take a holistic approach to treatment. This means that your treatment team emphasizes your involvement in your care. Your treatment team may include: physicians, psychologists, social workers, recreation specialists, nursing staff, art therapists, counselors and dietitians, each of whom respect the needs of the whole person. Your physical, emotional, social, spiritual, cultural, and intellectual needs are all considered in your individualized treatment planning.

All patients follow a structured schedule. Daily programming includes multidisciplinary therapy, specialized group therapies, and interaction with treatment staff and other patients. As your treatment plan is designed, you and your treatment team will identify an aftercare plan to help you continue your treatment following discharge. Our goal provides you with an effective set of "tools" which, if used, will help you live a fuller, more satisfying life.

We also understand that you may be feeling anxious about your treatment. This handbook is designed to provide you with information to help you feel more comfortable. It is a guide to acquaint you with our program and policies, and with your responsibilities while at ▬▬▬▬▬▬▬. Again, if you have any concerns regarding the information in this booklet, or your treatment in general, please let us know.

Sincerely,

The Eating Disorder Center Staff

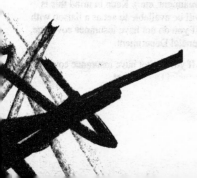

Our Mission

OUR PURPOSE is to be a premier provider of behavioral health care and associated services in a continuation of our near-century tradition.

WE BELIEVE in a skilled, professional team approach to individualized care within a treatment community, respecting the dignity and sanctity of each person.

OUR SUCCESS will be demonstrated through quality care, financial integrity, personal growth and community well being.

From the President

Thank you for choosing ▉▉▉▉▉▉▉▉▉▉▉ for your behavioral health needs. We hope that your stay with us will be beneficial. Even though the circumstances that brought you here may be difficult, you have found a safe place in which to seek support and comfort.

For nearly a century, we have been quietly offering hope, help and healing through comprehensive, quality care. We continually strive to provide the best services possible and we need your help to do so. Please feel free to complete a customer feedback form at any time during your stay so we can further enhance our quality of care.

Sincerely,

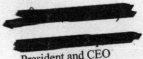

President and CEO

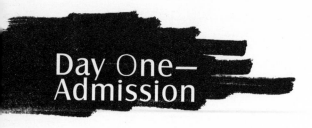

Day One— Admission

I step off the train at the Milwaukee depot, clutching my two battered suitcases and trying not to shake from anxiety and the diet pills I took during the ride. An older man with a grizzly gray beard is standing inside the dilapidated station with a sign that simply reads: NICOLE. I attempt to smile as I walk over to him.

"You Nicole?"

"Yes."

"Let's go, then."

I want to jump on one of the trains headed west, or east, or anywhere other than here.

The driver loads my suitcases into the white hospital van,

and I call my mother from my cell phone to let her know some-one picked me up at the train station. She wishes she could be here with me, but I am glad she is at home in Pennsylvania. I am embarrassed and don't want her to see me like this. I want to protect her from what I have become. The surly driver attempts to make conversation with me by identifying all the wildflowers along I-94 and telling me about his grandchildren. I only half listen to his ramblings and wonder if he thinks I'm thin enough to have an eating disorder. Finally, we pull up to the Eating Disorders Center (EDC). From the van, the EDC appears to be a rustic wooden structure surrounded by a carefully manicured and landscaped lawn. It does not look like a mental institution.

Residential Counselor (RC) Shannon meets me at the door. I notice immediately that she cannot be older than I am—her hair is too stylish; she says "like" when she talks—but I relegate that thought to the back of my mind. I am trying to keep an open mind about treatment. RC Shannon helps me wheel my suitcases into the office, where they will remain until she and RC Julia search them for contraband. Shannon hands me over to Mark, the person in charge of new-admission paperwork. He has numerous forms for me to sign and fill out.

I sign myself into the EDC, agree to pay any charges not covered by BlueCross BlueShield, agree to follow the hospital rules, sign a release allowing the psychiatrist to use my writing and artwork for his research, and fill out a survey to determine just how eating-disordered I truly am, and what eating disorder I have.

My first diagnosis is anorexia, binge/purge subtype, but it is later changed to EDNOS characterized by restriction and purging, since I'm not underweight and I still menstruate.

After I've signed all the forms, Mark shows me around the first floor of the EDC, where I will be a resident.

The EDC's interior is much like that of a college dorm, except for a few subtle differences. There are no locks on the bathroom or shower doors. The windows don't open without a special tool that is kept in the RC office, which resembles a nursing station in a medical hospital. The snack cupboards are locked, and the refrigerator door sports a formidable padlock. Then there are motivational posters, made by the residents during free time and art therapy, that are plastered all over any clear wall space: HUGS, NOT DRUGS; ONE DAY AT A TIME; YOU ARE BEAUTIFUL; EATING DISORDERS THRIVE IN THE DARK BUT DIE IN THE LIGHT. The Serenity Prayer is posted prominently on the wall as well.

I am trying very hard to rein in my sarcasm and negativity.

I find all this positive-attitude, recovery-speak propaganda to be utter bullshit.

Mark shows me the snack list taped to the cupboard door in the kitchenette. Each snack is assigned a certain number of exchanges according to its caloric content, and residents are assigned a number of exchanges to meet based on whether they are gaining or maintaining their weight. Cheerios bars (my favorite snack) are two exchanges. Oyster crackers are one exchange. Honey-wheat pretzels are three exchanges. This list of snacks and exchanges is overwhelming. My eyes widen and I look around for exits out of this positive-energy-laden place.

Then it is time for dinner. I wait in the dayroom with the other ten women who are residents on First Floor. Eliza, a petite woman who lives in the Twin Cities, is my age, and has blond dreadlocks introduces herself and takes me under her wing, asking me questions about myself and telling me about her personal history; for this I am grateful. Eliza is originally from Nebraska and struggles with alcoholism. In the following months, she and I will learn that we have much in common, and we will grow close. Courtney, a tall, thin woman is giggling on the sofa with Sarah, a short but shapely bleached blond whose style reminds me of Christina Aguilera's during her blond phase. A woman with dark brown hair and black-framed glasses curls into herself on the blue leather chair. I learn that she is Sandra from New York City, and that she is cross-addicted to heroin.

Someone named Laura, who is to be my roommate, is missing. She is in an individual session with Therapist Elaine. A pale, emaciated woman whose skin has a grayish cast bounces nervously on her toes, muttering to herself. I learn that mealtime makes Danielle, a purging anorexic, nervous. Holly, another resident from the Twin Cities, who is bulimic, does a crossword puzzle, then suddenly bellows, "It's time to feed the eating-disordered!" Everyone lines up in front of the locked dining room door, and I follow suit. I will learn that this is a ritual: Before every meal, Holly bellows her famous line and the RCs gather up the meal cards (records of our individual meal plans) and lead us into the dining room. I am left wondering how I will fit into this scattered group, with these women who are supposedly my peers, and who, like me, cannot seem to nourish themselves. All I know is that I am neither the thinnest nor the fattest in the group, which makes me feel better. Before I arrived at the EDC, I was terrified that I would be the largest resident, and that no one would believe I had an eating disorder.

RC Julia, a tall blond in khakis with a pronounced Wisconsin accent, unlocks the dining room door, and the other residents shuffle in and jostle each other for a view of the list of exchanges for tonight's meal. I hang back at the end of the line, nervously chomping on my ragged cuticles until they bleed and pushing stray pieces of my hair behind my ears. RC Julia and Eliza help me with my new-admission meal plan (the standard meal plan I'll have until I meet with the dietitian). I take one slice of ricotta-spinach pie, one carton of skim milk, and one mixed-fruit cup. RC Julia checks off my meal card; I have successfully met all my exchange requirements. As long as I eat all my food, I will be marked as "compliant." If I'm "incompliant," an RC will question my decision to not eat my food (not eating is symptomatic of a larger issue, according to the EDC staff). Incompliancy prevents a resident from moving up through the level system and gaining the privileges associated with each level.

I sit with RC Julia, Eliza, and another woman, who angrily slathers her bread with the required four tablespoons of peanut butter. RC Julia and Eliza try to talk to me, but I am petrified. This is too much food. Unless I can purge, I don't want to eat this much, and purging doesn't seem to be an option right now. Later, I will learn how to subvert the system, how to sneak down the hall and purge after meals, how to toss my snack off the deck and into the woods. But right now I am convinced that I have just signed away my right to an eating disorder.

I am shaking from the diet pills and Diet Coke I consumed on the train ride here. Otherwise, I have not eaten anything all day (my last hunger strike, what I believe will be my last act of eating-disordered defiance). I should be hungry right now, but I'm not. I will have to relearn hunger cues: when I'm hungry versus when I want to eat to fill some void within me, or when I'm symbolically purging myself of emotion via food.

I eat everything but the fruit cup. I know I could eat the fruit cup. The reduced-sugar fruit cups I allow myself to eat are seventy calories each and taste of artificial sweetener, but these fruit cups are not reduced sugar. I can taste the difference. I'm estimating the EDC fruit cup at ninety calories, but I still won't eat it, mostly out of protest, and because I'm convinced the ricotta-spinach pie is loaded with fat and calories. Secretly, I yearn for the slippery peach cubes, to scoop up the thick, golden nectar with my spoon and swish the sugary liquid around in my mouth, but doing so would be a sign of weakness, of giving in to my hunger.

RC Julia tells me I did a good job with my meal. My incompliancy is forgiven because the first meal is never easy for anyone. I think back to last week at this time. I was finishing up an essay for my Poetry of Social Change workshop and grading student papers. I was roaming around Minneapolis as I pleased. Now I'm sitting in an institution where someone practically my own age (RC Julia is twenty-three) is in charge of me and has just complimented me on eating most of my dinner.

After everyone has finished (or not finished) dinner, we file back into the dayroom and sit in a circle on worn and comfortable furniture. Each woman introduces herself, offers a little information about her history, and talks about how her day went. Then she sets goals for the next day and says whether or not she accomplished her goal for today. My introduction goes like this: "Hi, I'm Nicole, I'm twenty-two, I'm a graduate student in creative writing at the University of Minnesota, I'm originally from Pennsylvania, and this is my first time in treatment."

Everyone looks at me for a moment. They are waiting for the rest of the introduction.

"And I have a mom, a dad, a brother, a dog, and a cat."

I think the second part of the introduction is absolutely ridiculous. It sounds like a kindergarten exercise. Later, I will refuse to say that I have a mom, a dad, a brother, a dog, and a cat. But I don't want to get in trouble within hours of arriving at the EDC, so I go along with it.

"What is your goal for tomorrow?" asks RC Julia.

"To get adjusted and settle in."

One of the EDC nurses pokes her head into the dayroom and

asks if she can get a medical history on me. I follow her to the conference room and answer her seemingly endless questions.

"Health problems, other than the eating disorder?"

"Asthma and heart problems."

"What kind of heart problems?"

"PVCs, PACs, and bradycardia."

The nurse records all this information on her computer without blinking. She is used to hearing about eating disorder–induced heart problems. She takes my temperature.

"Ninety-seven point zero—that's low."

"I always run a bit low."

"Eating disorder patients often have lower temperatures, pulse rates, and blood pressure."

Next, she takes my blood pressure. As the cuff inflates on my arm, I know this won't be good. My blood pressure is usually low, even when I'm healthy. Lately, though, it has been abnormally low.

"Ninety over sixty—that's low. Now I need you to stand up so I can take your pressure again and see if it drops."

I stand up. My blood pressure drops to 80/53. This explains my frequent dizziness when I wake up in the morning, and why everything turns black and sparkly if I don't stand up slowly. This condition is called orthostasis. The nurse assigns me mandatory blood pressure checks every morning. If I drop below 80/40, I'll be put on a special watch.

I tell the nurse about my drug allergies (Ceclor, Septra, Compazine, Claritin-D); my hospitalizations (tonsillectomy at age four;

concussion, dehydration, and irregular heartbeat at twenty-two); my current medications (multivitamin, Zyrtec); my menstrual cycles (almost nonexistent since I lost weight); how much weight I've lost in the past year (approximately thirty pounds); how often I purge (sometimes once a day, sometimes multiple times a day, at least five times a week); the brand and number of diet pills I take (Metabolife or Dexatrim, upward of two a day); my caloric consumption (no more than five hundred calories per day, or I have to purge and take extra diet pills); how long I've had an eating disorder (since I was thirteen). The nurse tells me that I'm scheduled to be driven into town the next day for a physical from Dr. Lorensky, who examines every EDC patient within twenty-four hours of arrival. Then she draws a few vials of blood to check my CBCs and electrolytes. After she draws my blood, she asks me to pee in a cup so she can check my urine for infection, ketones, and evidence of drug use.

After I meet with the nurse, RC Julia and RC Shannon pull me aside and tell me it's time to search my suitcases. We go into my room, and they each take a suitcase. I feel violated as RC Julia paws through my underwear and searches my bras for contraband. RC Shannon flips quickly through my journal, and I resist the urge to tear it from her hands.

RC Julia and RC Shannon are respectful. They refold all my clothes and are gentle with my papers. They make small talk with me the whole time. RC Julia goes through my purse, pulls out my bottle of diet pills, and takes them to the office to be disposed of. Then it is all over, and I'm left in my room with my suitcases. I set to putting away my things, even though I don't think I will be here long, because I have convinced myself that my eating disorder will be under control by my birthday, at the end of June.

Laura, my assigned roommate, throws open the door and flings herself onto her unmade bed. I have surmised that she is crazy. Not crazy in an *I consume five thousand calories in one sitting and then stick my finger down my throat and vomit* way, but in an *I'm obsessed with serial killers and I've spent serious time in lockdown* way. Laura is wearing fatigue pants and a pale pink camisole that showcases her prominent collarbone. She asks if I want the "grand tour" and stares me down with intense brown eyes. I say yes. She shows me which drawers and what closet are to be mine, and where I can store my things in the bathroom.

Laura tells me she is from South Carolina and is a purging anorexic, meaning that anything she eats, she usually throws up. Prior to coming to the EDC, she did a stint in detox (Laura is also an alcoholic and a drug addict; cross-addiction is common among ED patients), and then went to a treatment program in Utah, where she was kicked out for alcohol possession.

RC Shannon comes into our room and tells me I have to take my nighttime meds and get a picture taken for my chart, for identification purposes. I follow her to the office, where I tell her and RC Julia that I don't take any medication, other than a multivitamin and allergy medication in the morning.

RC Shannon asks me to smile so she can take my picture. The flash goes off and the camera spits out an image. My expression is somewhere between a frown and a grimace. My diet pills have just been confiscated, I'm not allowed to have Diet Coke, I'm not allowed to purge, and I have just eaten something called ricotta-spinach pie. I see no reason to smile.

RC Julia tells me it's snack time.

I'm still full from dinner but take a red apple from the refrigerator. I don't like red apples, I like only green apples, but everything else seems too risky to eat without the possibility of purging. I eat one-quarter of my apple and show the remainder of the apple to RC Julia before I pitch it into the trash. She doesn't give me a hard time about not finishing my snack, and I decide that I like her.

Holly stumbles into the office, claiming she has just purged blood in the bathroom. Her face is pale, and she lies down in the hallway because she is afraid she will pass out. RC Julia calls an ambulance while RC Shannon takes Holly's blood pressure. It registers at 40/10. Laura and Sandra hold Holly's hands and tell her help is on the way. The ambulance crew files up the stairs and straps Holly onto the stretcher. At the local hospital (the EDC is part of a psychiatric hospital), nurses and doctors suction blood out of Holly's stomach as she fades in and out of consciousness. She has a Mallory-Weiss tear, which is a tear in her esophageal lining from the strain of her constant purging. Holly returns the next morning, after countless IV bags of saline and potassium. The tear should heal if she stops purging and takes her gastric medication.

During this drama, the other residents watch music videos on VH-1 (it's the summer of Britney Spears, OutKast, and Christina

Aguilera), smoke on the deck, or talk on their cell phones. Holly is prone to health crises, so her purging blood does not shock anyone. RC Julia assures me that an ambulance crew at the EDC is a rarity. I decide to comment on some of my students' papers at the back table. I put my headphones on and listen to Tom Petty's *Wildflowers* album while I comment. I am inside my head, and I am trying as best I can to forget that I am at the EDC. As long as I'm working on things pertaining to school, I can hold on to the person I am outside these institutional walls.

I sit at the back table, absorbed in commenting, until 10:00 PM, when I decide to go to bed. In the morning, I will be weighed facing backward so I can't see my weight. My blood pressure will be dangerously low. I will find out that my potassium is low and will start a regimen of potassium tablets that will last long after my discharge, and I will learn that I have a vitamin deficiency. Tonight I sleep the sleep of the exhausted, curled up on my regulation hospital bed, on thin, white institutional sheets with a flat pillow, wondering how I ended up in this place.

Psychiatric Evaluation

tient is a 22-year-old,
gle white female in
asters program in
ative writing at the
iversi
lly fr

Patient is a 22-year-old, single, white female in Masters Program in Creative Writing at the University of Minnesota, originally from Pennsylvania.

"I'm eating-disordered." Patient describes onset of purging at age 14 with original issue being difficulty of adjusting to onset of puberty associated with weight changes. Things worsened when she went to boarding school at age 16. Patient says binges "atypical." Typical binge is a candy bar. Typical pattern would be purging 3x a week. No purging from April to September of the past year, but things have progressively worsened over the academic year, with stress. Low weight 117 at 17 years old. High weight 160, now weighs

133 with decrease this year. Also restricts, less than 1,000 calories a day, skips meals, no meat. Takes diet pills, denies laxatives and diuretics. Denies compulsive exercise.

Treatment has included individual psychotherapy and eating disorder group that patient did not attend regularly due to school conflict.

In Jan/Feb, patient had episode of syncope, related concussion, electrolyte abnormality and heart rhythm irregularity.

Patient denies any problems with depression and related symptoms although sleep is irregular. Some anxiety, she feels may be related to diet pills.

No prior psychiatric hospitalization. Some self-injury when 12 or 13, related to poor school performance. Trial of Paxil, 20 mgs for 1 year to help binge/purge cycle when 17–19. Did not feel right—sedated.

Social drinker.

Episode of syncope and concussion, heart rhythm irregularities in the form of PVCs, PACs and bradycardia. Exercise-induced asthma. Ovarian cysts. Seasonal allergies.

Allergies: Ceclor, Septra, Compazine, Claritin-d.

From intact family. Oldest child. 16-year-old brother at boarding school. Parents not college-educated, was pressure for patient to do well in school and patient feels this relates to perfectionist qualities. Father is an operations manager. Mother is an accountant. Enjoyed boarding school. Switched from Ohio University to Penn State Erie where she got BA. History of dating, most recent relationship female. Has been barely functional at the U of M.

Appropriate hygiene, good eye contact, speech normal, "some anxiety here," affect full.

Anorexia, binge/purge subtype. History of eating disorder since age 14, characterized by bingeing and purging or restricting. Patient relates perfectionist traits and poor body image as a related issue. No prominent disruption in mood at this point.

No psychiatric medications at this point.

Day Two—
Weight and Vitals

I am awakened at six o'clock that first morning, when Natalie,
the night-shift residential counselor, opens the door and chirps, in a
singsong kindergarten-teacher voice, "Time for weight and vitals!"

Sunlight filters through the blinds and casts patterns on the
white sheet. I lie there for a moment, stretch my arms over my head,
and stand up. On a bad morning, I will mutter, "Fuckin' Natalie,"
pull the covers over my head, and refuse weight and vitals. But I
decide that I will try to make my first morning a good one, although
I dread stepping on the scale and not knowing my weight, that mea-
surement that has defined so many of my days for so long.
Natalie is one of the most obese people I have ever met (staff

thinks this is why most residents despise her—she is what we think we will be if we stop starving and barfing), and every night she brings a smorgasbord of fast food with her to the EDC, to binge on while we sleep. Natalie's arms are swathed in duct tape bandages. Sandra asks Natalie why she adorns her arms in duct tape, and we find out Natalie has warts, which seems fitting. Natalie is a compulsive overeater. Compulsive overeating is an eating disorder that is treated at the EDC. Yet staff has hired Natalie to watch over all of us almost every night of the week (on her nights off, RC Shannon usually fills in).

In my closet is a drafty, standard-issue hospital gown. I take off my pajama pants and tank top, ball them up, and toss them on the bed. Before wrapping the gown around myself, I do a body check, taking inventory of my breasts, waist, hips, and thighs, making sure nothing has changed since the night before, that none of my parts have expanded. Some days I stand naked in front of the mirror and I swear I can see the fat cells thickening my waist. We are allowed to wear underwear and a gown when we are getting weighed, but we cannot wear slippers.

The hall lights are bright and I squint as I shuffle down the hall, clad in slippers and gown, arms crossed over my chest because we may not wear a bra during weight and vitals (the metal underwire might boost our weight).

Other residents are stumbling bleary-eyed down the hall. Many of them appear haunted. There is no luster to their skin, and their eyes are sunk in deep, hollow sockets. This early-morning scene, when I am not quite awake, is surreal. It's as if I am floating through a land of apparitions.

Natalie, in her duct-taped glory, is waiting for me.

A pink binder with my name on the spine is sitting on the table in the office. Natalie has it opened to my weight-and-vitals page. I sit down on an uncomfortable office chair and extend my right arm and open my mouth when she asks me to do so. She slides the thermometer under my tongue and wraps the blood pressure cuff around my arm.

This will become a source of contention for me. Natalie uses the child-size cuff, which I will dub the anorexic cuff. I am not underweight, and therefore do not need the anorexic cuff. An adult cuff would work just fine, but Natalie will insist on using the anorexic cuff, even though it will burst off my strangulated arm on a regular basis. RC Julia will tell me to "use my voice" and confront Natalie about using the wrong blood pressure cuff. I will tell RC Julia that I want to avoid the prospect of any conversation with Natalie. I will tend to peer at her with sleep-slit eyes in the morning, and when she asks how I slept, I will grunt.

After taking my temperature, blood pressure, and pulse, Natalie weighs me. She turns on the scale and has me take off my slippers, turn around, and step on backward so I don't see my weight. After the scale beeps I step off, put my slippers back on, and head back to my room to wake up Laura (no small task, since she is on massive amounts of tranquilizers, antidepressants, antipsychotics, and sleeping meds) and get ready for the inevitable: breakfast.

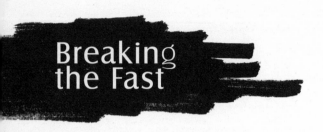

Breaking
the Fast

lly bellows her infamous
e.

Holly bellows her infamous line, and RC Erica and RC Allison
lead us into the dining room for breakfast. Everyone but me and
the RCs is still in pajamas. I soon learn that no one bothers to
change out of pajamas unless we're leaving the EDC. Why mope
around in jeans when you can mope around just as well, if not
better, in loose-fitting pajama pants and a sweatshirt? But that first
morning, I wear the jeans I wore on the train the day before, as
well as a fitted black V-neck shirt. My hair hangs around my face,
and I try to hide behind it as much as possible.

In the food line, I pick out one English muffin, two packets of
butter, a fruit cup, and a carton of skim milk. Back at the table, RC

Allison introduces herself and checks that I have met my exchange requirements. Perhaps she senses that I am struggling as I stare at the food on my plate, trying desperately not to cry, throw the plate at the wall, or run screaming into the woods of southeast Wisconsin. RC Allison sets her plate down on the table and begins buttering her toast as she asks me where I'm from and where I go to school. I answer in monosyllables and play with my peach chunks.

I observe RC Allison furtively. She is a pale redhead with blue eyes, and I think she is pretty. *This is what healthy women look like,* I tell myself. RC Allison's eyes are not sunk into her skull, her hair shines a bright copper under the lights, and her skin is smooth and clear in a way that mine is not. RC Allison does not play with her food—she simply eats it—and this amazes me.

Eliza and Laura are the two other women at my table. Laura bolts out of her chair as soon as she finishes eating, and heads to the deck that is adjacent to the dining room to have her post-breakfast cigarette. Eliza lingers over a cup of herbal tea and talks to me and RC Allison while I slowly eat my English muffin. RC Allison tells us about Anthony, her fiancé, who is in the military. She tells us about her dogs and gives me a crash course in what southeast Wisconsin is like. Both RC Allison and Eliza ask me about growing up in Pennsylvania, but I can't concentrate on talking to them about Pennsylvania while I'm trying to eat.

Eventually, I gulp down the last drop of my milk and RC Allison marks me as compliant. I discard my tray and join the smokers on the deck because we are not allowed to be alone for two hours after meals and one hour after snack, since we might sneak down the hall and purge or attempt to exercise off the food we just ate. So I stand on the deck with the other residents and wait for whatever happens next.

Dr. Lorensky

After breakfast, Mark informs me that he will drive me into town to get a physical. I assume I am the only resident going, but when I walk out to the van, I see another resident sulking in the back seat. I'm wearing black pajama pants, tennis shoes, and my Penn State sweatshirt because I am exhausted. This is my first day without caffeine, diet pills, and purging, and I am struggling to stay awake and alert. My limbs are heavy and I have a pounding headache. I almost pass out every time I stand up, but I fight the black sparkly stars because I don't want to be sent to the hospital. Breakfast sits in my stomach, although the English muffin, skim milk, and fruit cup I ate keep lunging up my throat. My stomach is trying to evict them.

Before she released me to Mark, RC Allison handed me a packet of graham crackers for my morning snack. I am to eat the graham crackers and then show the empty wrapper to Mark, who will report back to RC Allison. I trudge, graham crackers in hand, to the van. I say hello to the pale, gaunt teenager from the adolescent floor in the back seat as I climb in. She glares at me and clutches a snack-size box of raisins. When Mark isn't looking, she stuffs the raisins under the seat in front of her and shows Mark the empty box. He nods and throws the raisin box into a plastic trash bag.

We stop at the obsessive-compulsive disorder (OCD) cottage to pick up an OCD resident. The resident is a young woman in her twenties who appears to be on the verge of a massive anxiety attack. Her eyes dart left and right, left and right. I smile at her and she tries to smile back at me, but her lips just quiver.

At Dr. Lorensky's office, Mark announces that we are here for our admission physicals. An old man reading *National Geographic* peers at us from behind his bifocals, and I want to sink into the gray industrial carpet beneath my feet. I have officially been adjudicated as crazy. Before I can blush bright red, a nurse calls my name.

She smiles a perfunctory nurse smile and asks me to step on the scale backward. I oblige. I hear the click of the metal balancers sliding along the numbered bar. After she weighs me, she leads me to an exam room, where she records my drug allergies and takes my blood pressure and temperature, both of which are low, per usual.

Dr. Lorensky marches into the room. She's a formidable Polish woman with a stiff helmet of bleached hair. She listens to my heart and notes my dismal pulse. She shakes her head and asks about the diet pills, purging, and caffeine. She checks the glands under my chin for swelling. They're swollen from purging.

I lie down on my back and she presses on my stomach. As I unbutton the top of my jeans she notices my tan line.

"Been to the beach lately?" she asks.

"Just the tanning booth," I say.

"That causes cancer," she says.

"I know."

"Your health is a mess."

"I know."

Dr. Lorensky spends the better part of a half hour preaching at me and scolding me about my apparent disregard for my health. She requests a repeat EKG and the results of my cardiology workup in Minnesota. By the time I leave her office, I am waiting for my potassium-deficient heart to seize up on me, for my diet-pill-induced overactive thyroid to cause my eyes to bulge out of my head, and for a suspicious mole on my arm to metastasize into a particularly virulent strain of malignant melanoma. I wonder if this visit to Dr. Lorensky is part of my recovery plan (scare the patient into recovery), and if the EDC is like the army in that it is going to break me down and then build me back up.

Yet, a year after I am discharged from the EDC, I receive my medical records and discover that Dr. Lorensky found me to be a "well-nourished, well-developed young woman," despite her diagnosis of low potassium, low and orthostatic blood pressure, low thyroid-stimulating hormone, dizziness/fainting, anorexia, and bulimia.

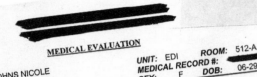

MEDICAL EVALUATION

UNIT: EDI ROOM: 512-A
MEDICAL RECORD #: █████
SEX: F DOB: 06-29-1981

PATIENT NAME: JOHNS NICOLE
ADMIT DATE: 05-24-2004
ATTD. PHYSICIAN: █████

CHIEF COMPLAINT: Eating disorder.

HISTORY OF PRESENT ILLNESS: The patient is a 22-year-old, Caucasian female admitted to the Residential Eating Disorder Program a few days ago for treatment of anorexia and bulimia. She restricts, and she purges up to five times a week. She denies laxative or diuretic use, but she uses metabolite 2 tablets daily. She suffers from an eating disorder on and off since age 14. She also over exercises, she says she runs for 1 ½ hours daily. She lost 30 pounds since September of last year.

ALLERGIES: She is allergic to Ceclor, sulfa, Compazine, Claritin D and Ilosone. She also suffers from seasonal allergies.

CURRENT MEDICATIONS: Zyrtec 10 mg daily, Maxair inhaler p.r.n., potassium supplement, ibuprofen p.r.n., EpiPen p.r.n., Benadryl p.r.n.

PAST MEDICAL HISTORY: (1) She had an anaphylactic reaction once in the past to unknown source; she carried an EpiPen with her. (2) Exercise-induced asthma. (3) Hospitalized in January or February of this year due to near syncopal episode. She also had an irregular heartbeat, PVC's, orthostatic hypotension, bradycardia, and abnormal electrolytes. She has been followed by a cardiologist. She states that her echocardiogram and Holter monitor both were within normal limits. (4) She denies history of diabetes, hypertension, hyperlipidemia, seizures, anemia, blood dyscrasias, or any other medical problems or surgeries other than mentioned above. (5) Tonsillectomy and adenoidectomy.

FAMILY HISTORY: Mother suffers from hypothyroidism. Father is alive and well. The patient has a 16-year-old brother who is healthy. Maternal grandmother has hypothyroidism and the rest of her grandparents are in good health.

SOCIAL HISTORY: She does not smoke, she drinks alcohol only socially, and she never used any illicit drugs. She graduated from the University of Minnesota.

REVIEW OF SYSTEMS: She complains of intermittent dizziness and lightheadedness. Denies any headache or blurred vision. Denies any earache, sore throat, or sinus congestion. Denies fever, chills, or productive cough. Denies chest pain, palpitations, shortness of breath, or pedal edema. Denies hematemesis and melena. Denies chest pain, nausea, vomiting, diarrhea, but complains of constipation. Denies vaginal discharge or bleeding. The patient's last menstrual period was two or three weeks ago and her periods are most of the time regular. Denies urinary frequency, dysuria, or hematuria. Denies any numbness or paresthesias. Denies any back problem. Denies joint pain or swelling. polydipsia, polyuria, or heat or cold intolerance.

PHYSICAL EXAMINATION: Physical examination reveals a young, well-developed, well-nourished, Caucasian female with the following vital signs. Temperature is ___°. Pulse is 60 and regular. Blood pressure is 90/74. Respirations are 16. She is 5 feet 4 3/4 inches tall and weighs 134 pounds.

Skin: The skin appeared to be normal in color and texture. There were no obvious serious eruptions. The mucous membranes were moist. There were no obvious areas of discoloration or pigmentation. There was no evidence of jaundice or cyanosis. The texture of the hair was normal and the distribution of the hair over the body was normal. There was no telangiectasis present. There were no obvious areas of petechiae or ecchymosis.

PATIENT NAME: JOHNS NICOLE
REPORT: MEDICAL EVALUATION

MEDICAL RECORD
ADMIT DATE: 05-24-2004

Head: The head was normocephalic. There were no masses noted. Hair distribution was normal. There were no obvious scars or deformities. The condition of the scalp appeared to be normal. There was no evidence of tenderness or bony exostosis.

Face: There was no evidence of paralysis or abnormal movements about the face. There were no areas of tenderness or swelling.

Eyes: The pupils were round and equal and react to light directly and consensually. The sclera and conjunctiva were free of jaundice. All extraocular movements were normal. The cornea did not appear to be opaque. The lids showed no evidence of petechia.

Funduscopic exam: Normal ocular fundi. Optic disc borders are distinct and clear with no evidence of bulging or cupping of the optic discs. There was no A-V nicking. There was no evidence of hemorrhages or exudates.

Ears: Hearing appears to be grossly intact. There is no evidence of discharge within the external auditory meati. The tympanic membranes appeared to be normal, intact with no inflammation and have a normal light reflex. There were no posterior auricular nodes present.

Nose: There was no evidence of nasal discharge or inflammation. There was no evidence of obstruction or polyps. The septum was midline. The nasal turbinates appeared to be normal and there was no evidence of sinus tenderness on palpation.

Mouth: The gums appeared to be of normal color and were without lesions. The tongue was midline and did not deviate. The hydration appeared to be normal. The tongue papillae appeared to be normal in size, shape, and distribution. There was no evidence of fasciculation. There were no lesions noted on the tongue. Buccal mucosa appeared pink and moist.

Throat: The uvula was in the midline. The palate appeared to be normal. There were no exudates or inflammation.

Neck: The neck was supple and mobile with no nuchal rigidity. The trachea was in the midline. There was no palpable adenopathy. The thyroid was not palpable. There was no jugular-venous distention.

Chest: The thorax appeared to be symmetrical in size and shape. The diaphragm appeared to expand normally and equally on each side. There was no tenderness on the palpitation of the thorax.

Lungs: The lungs were clear to auscultation. There were no audible wheezes, rales, or rhonchi.

Heart: Auscultation revealed a normal sinus rhythm with no gallops, murmurs, or extra sounds.

Abdomen: Inspection of the abdomen revealed the size and contour to be normal. There was no evidence of dilated veins or visible peristalsis. Palpation of the abdomen revealed no evidence of spasm, tenderness, rigidity, guarding, and masses. There were no hernias palpated.

Extremities: Peripheral pulses were bilaterally equal and strong. There were no clubbing, cyanosis, or edema.

MEDICAL RECORD #:
ADMIT DATE: 05-24-2004

PATIENT NAME: JOHNS NICOLE
REPORT: MEDICAL EVALUATION

Neurological exam: Cranial nerves II - Peripheral vision and visual fields appear grossly intact. Optic disk was visualized and appeared normal without cupping or bulging, and the disk borders appear distinct and clear. Cranial nerves III, IV, and VI - Extraocular movements appear to be grossly intact in all directions. The pupils were round and equal and respond to light directly and consensually. Cranial nerve V - Facial sensations appear to be intact. Cranial nerve VII - Symmetrical facial movements were noted. Cranial nerve VIII - Hearing appeared to be grossly intact. Cranial IX, X, XI, and XII - Voice appeared normal. Tongue movements were normal without any focal signs. Swallowing was present without difficulty. Motor exam reveals no focal atrophy. No obvious weakness was noted. No asymmetrical tone was noted. Deep tendon reflexes appeared bilaterally equal and brisk. There were no resting tremors. Finger-to-nose testing was intact with and without the eyes open. There was no asterixis. The Romberg was negative. The gait was normal tandem.

Basically this is a normal examination.

LABORATORY DATA: Her TSH is low at 0.07. Her glucose is 96. BUN 7. Creatinine 0.8, SGOT 21, SGPT 41, alkaline phosphatase 82, total bilirubin 0.8, calcium 9.3, phosphorus 4.2, magnesium 1.9, total protein 6.9, albumin 4.1, sodium 140, potassium 3.3, chloride 103. White count is 5.1, hemoglobin 14.8, hematocrit 40.7, platelet count 188, normal differential.

IMPRESSION:
1. Low TSH.
2. Hypokalemia.
3. Hypotension.
4. Dizziness most likely due to orthostatic hypotension.
5. Eating disorder.

PLAN: Her potassium was supplemented with oral K-Dur and it will be repeated periodically. Her TSH and free T4 will be repeated next week. Will check orthostatic blood pressure and will encourage increased fluid intake. I will follow her medically while she is here.

Observation

After my visit to Dr. Lorensky, I spend the rest of my first full day at the EDC napping on the sofa and meeting various members of my treatment team. For the first seventy-two hours, every EDC resident is restricted to the floor, as most women arrive somewhat medically unstable. The first full day is a blur of memories: I remember eating a snack and meals when told to eat, standing up and almost passing out several times, falling into a deep, dreamless state that was more coma than sleep, and meeting with Therapist Elaine and Dietitian Caroline.

Therapist Elaine tells me I filled out my patient survey with the most attention to detail she has ever seen. I take this as a compliment. I tell her about my eating-disordered behaviors, about my childhood, my life in Minnesota, and other necessary facts. Perhaps what I don't tell her is most significant, but at this point I simply don't trust Therapist Elaine or anyone else at the EDC. I am guarded. In time, I will decide how much of my history to divulge. But for now, I am suspicious of this perky young woman with bright green eyes and a Wisconsin accent that rivals RC Julia's.

Dietitian Caroline tells me that most residents hate her, and that their hatred is completely understandable and normal, as she decides our meal plan. As I listen to Dietitian Caroline, I wonder how anyone can hate this woman with the gentle voice and empathetic eyes.

"Would you like to know how much you weighed this morning, Nicole?"

"Yes, please."

I am hoping Caroline does not hear the desperation in my voice.

"You weighed 131.5. We're setting your target weight range at 127–140. Does that sound reasonable?"

"Yes," I say.

Secretly, my brain is screaming, *Fuck, no.* The thought of weighing 140 again gets me panicking. I start to sweat and am fighting back tears. I begin to wonder if it's too late to back out, to sign myself out and leave this place, with its meal plans and weight ranges. I have fought to lose every single fucking pound, and I do not want to gain it back. Every pound lost was a battle, an exertion of willpower and strength. I wear my now-loose jeans like a badge of courage and proudly display my newfound clavicle. I run my hands over the fine bones of my ribs and cup my hipbones delicately, tracing the sharp outline with my index finger. I stare lovingly at my now-defined jaw in the mirror. I have liberated my jawline from the double chins that used to occupy it.

I am at war with my body.

When my scale blinked 127 at me, I jumped and whooped with elation. Only seventeen more pounds until I was officially underweight, and underweight was my ultimate goal, because then I could start over—my body would be reduced to its bare essentials, and everything would be okay.

"Nicole, what are you thinking about?" asks Dietitian Caroline.

"Nothing, I'm just tired," I lie.

"Well, you can go nap if you like," says Dietitian Caroline.

I try to nap, but underneath my blanket I frantically run my hands up and down the xylophone bones of my rib cage in an effort to reassure myself that I am not fat.

That night, all the residents except Holly and me go on an outing to Milwaukee. I can't go because I'm on observation, and Holly can't go because she purged blood last night. Since the RCs on First Floor are accompanying the residents on the outing, Holly and I have to stay on Lower Level while they are gone. We trudge down the stairs and take over one of the Lower Level sofas and watch *American Idol*. Holly texts in her vote for Kelly Clarkson, and I am bored and dreading snack time. The Lower Level is composed of older women and adolescent boys, a strange combination. I write in my journal and attempt to watch television. Eventually, I venture out to the back porch and call some of my friends from my cell phone, but no one is home. Holly comes out to join me, lights a cigarette, and offers me one, which I accept.

"Where are you from again?" she asks.

"Pennsylvania."

"Oh yeah, that's right, but you go to the University of Minnesota, right?"

"Yeah, but I don't think I'm going back. I hate it there."

"Are you some kind of genius or something? You're in graduate school and you're only twenty-two?" she asks with a grin.

"No, I'm not a genius," I reply, thinking about how I am the lousiest writer in the program, probably because I spend more time barfing than writing.

"I had to drop out of school a bunch of times; I'm still a sophomore in college," says Holly.

"Yeah, I thought I was going to have to drop out this past semester," I say.

"Most everyone here has dropped at least one semester of college. It's kind of hard to stay focused on school when you're so sick with the eating disorder," says Holly.

I exhale smoke out of my mouth and try not to cough, while Holly blows smoke out her nose and laughs at my amateur smoking attempts.

RC Marie calls Holly and me in for evening snack. Holly picks pretzels and I pick cheddar Chex Mix. RC Marie introduces herself;

I am suspicious of her pleasant temperament. She sits beside me on the sofa and tells me about her baby girl and asks me how I'm adjusting to EDC life. Later, RC Marie tells me she thought I was shy, as did most of the EDC staff, because I said so little in my first days there. Really, I was just too overwhelmed and too sick to string together many coherent thoughts. RC Marie excuses herself, saying she has to go pump, and I am confused about what she is pumping until Holly tells me RC Marie is breastfeeding.

When the First Floor residents return from the outing, Holly and I go back upstairs, now friends after our cigarette break. It's time for nighttime meds, and then it's off to sleep again.

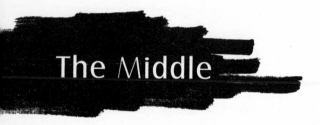

The Middle

sclaimer the middle is essy.

Disclaimer: The middle is messy.

The summer has a sense of timelessness, as day after regimented day fades into another. We, as EDC residents, are no longer part of the world. Instead, we are part of an insular microcosm where the rules are defined and enforced. New arrivals bring the breath of the outside world, the "real world," as we dub it. Then they, too, fade into our routine. We are all very tired. Our damaged bodies are attempting to mend, and our minds are exhausted from therapy. Any venture into the real world leaves us fatigued. There are food courts to avoid, traffic to deal with, and evidence that most people are living their lives. We sleep during any free moment. I fall into such a deep sleep during my late-afternoon naps that I liken them to comas.

I awaken disoriented and confused about where I am. Then I remember.

Phone calls from the outside world are an intrusion, as are visitors. We form unique bonds among ourselves—we are a sort of Sisterhood of the Starving, and we are our own society, complete with hierarchies and rank. Each of us has a function within the group. We pretend to hate the staff, our guardians. In loco parentis. Secretly, we love them. They protect us from our self-destruction.

What is Normal Eating?

Normal eating is going to the table hungry and eating until you are satisfied. It is being able to choose food you like and eat it and truly get enough of it–not just stop eating because you think you should. Normal eating is being able to give some thought to your food selection so you get nutritious food, but not being so wary and restrictive that you miss out on enjoyable food. Normal eating is giving yourself permission to eat sometimes because you are happy, sad, or bored, or just because it feels good. Normal eating is three meals a day, or four or five, or it can be choosing to munch along the way. It is leaving some cookies on the plate because you know you can have some again tomorrow, or it is eating more now because they taste so wonderful. Normal eating is overeating at times, feeling stuffed and uncomfortable. And it can be undereating at times and wishing you had more. Normal eating is trusting your body to make up for your mistakes in eating. Normal eating takes up some of your time and attention, but keeps its place as only one important area of your life.

In short, normal eating is flexible. It varies in response to your hunger, your schedule, your proximity to food, and your feelings.

It is easy to place blame. My father calls me one night; I know he's been reading books about how to help his eating-disordered daughter when he asks me if I've figured out the root cause of my eating disorder. If only it were that simple. Our gut impulse: Blame the media, blame the parents.

It's not so simple.

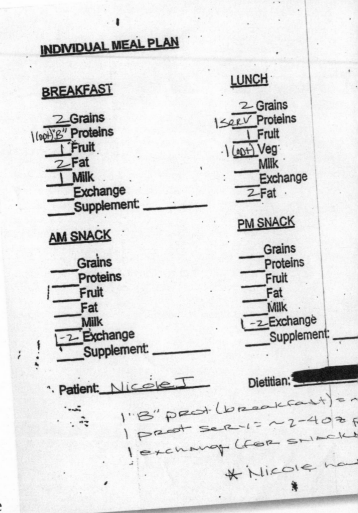

INDIVIDUAL MEAL PLAN

BREAKFAST

2 Grains
1 (oot) "B" Proteins
1 Fruit
2 Fat
1 Milk
___ Exchange
___ Supplement: _____

AM SNACK

___ Grains
___ Proteins
1 Fruit
___ Fat
___ Milk
1-2 Exchange
___ Supplement: _____

LUNCH

2 Grains
1 serv Proteins
1 Fruit
1 (oot) Veg
___ Milk
___ Exchange
2 Fat

PM SNACK

___ Grains
___ Proteins
___ Fruit
___ Fat
___ Milk
1-2 Exchange
___ Supplement: _____

Patient: Nicole J   Dietitian: ▓▓▓▓▓

1 "B" prot (breakfast) = ~
1 prot serv = ~2-40z f
1 exchange (for snack
   * Nicole ha

What is the purpose of **YOUR** meal plan?

1. to maintain my weight
2. to eat a balanced diet
3. to eat regularly so I don't have binge urges
4. to give me energy
5. to keep me healthy

What will make **YOU** a success with **YOUR** meal plan (now and after discharge)?

1. actually following it as closely as possible.
2. not always eating the same foods.
3. being okay w/ slight deviations.
4. being willing to try new things
5. not restricting bc it sets me up for a binge.
6. not cutting out exchanges.
7. eating at a regular set time
8. not taking diet pills or abusing caffeine to numb hunger.
9. not eating emotionally
10. listening to my body's internal cues.

DATE: 8-13-04

DINNER

__2__ Grains
__1 serv__ Proteins
__1__ Fruit
__1 (opt)__ Veg
____ Milk
____ Exchange
__2__ Fat

HS SNACK

____ Grains
____ Proteins
____ Fruit
____ Fat
____ Milk
__1-2__ Exchange
____ Supplement: _____

Calorie Level: _____

prot

kcal / exchange

on self select

73

Meal Plans

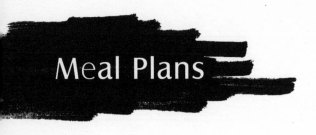

BREAKFAST:

2 grains (1 English muffin)

akfast lunch dinner snacks

2 fats (2 packets of butter)

1 fruit (banana)

1 milk (carton of skim)

LUNCH/DINNER:

2 grains (2 slices of bread)

2 fats (2 packets of butter)

2 proteins (2 slices of turkey)

1 fruit (banana)

SNACKS:

3 (optional)

This is the customized meal plan Dietitian Caroline creates
for me after our initial meeting. It's a maintenance meal plan,
meaning I don't have to gain any weight, so I am spared the extra
calories of an Ensure supplement or nightly feedings adminis-
tered through a nasogastric feeding tube.[1] But I gain weight on
my maintenance meal plan, and this makes me hate my body
even more. Dietitian Caroline tells me that some of the weight
gain is due to my body's rehydrating itself, that some of it is
simply because my vital organs are replenishing themselves, but I
don't believe her.

Dietitian Caroline calls gaining up to eleven pounds while at
the EDC "maintaining." As the numbers creep up, I grow uncomfortable thinking about the burgeoning fat cells expanding my
thighs. My body is growing soft and fleshy. I am Rubenesque. I
am taking up too much space. My favorite jeans grow tighter, until
one day in early June I simply can't wear them anymore.

After one week at the EDC, I lie down in the hall and writhe
around on the floor because anger is coursing through my body and
I need to manifest my pain physically. Eliza asks what I am doing,

and I tell her my jeans are too tight. RC Julia watches this scene unfold from her chair in the office.

"You are really crawling out of your skin, Nicole."

"That's a really astute observation, Julia."

"You have to fight that eating disorder voice in your head."

"I'm fucking tired of fighting; I just want to fit into my jeans again."

1. A nasogastric feeding tube is a thin plastic tube inserted through the nose, past the throat, and down into the stomach, and through which Ensure can be pumped slowly into the patient over a course of a night. This helps speed the weight-gaining process and is usually used if a patient is severely underweight or medically unstable, or refuses to eat.

SNACK EXCHANGES
OCTOBER 2003

FOOD ITEM	PORTION	EXCHANGES
2 % Milk	1 carton	2 exchanges
Apple – green	1 each	1 exchange
Apple – red	1 each	1 exchange
Apple Juice	1 container (4 oz)	1 exchange
Baked Lays: Potato Chips	1 bag	2 exchanges
Baked Lays: Doritos	1 bag	3 exchanges
Cheddar Cheese Popcorn	1 bag	2 exchanges
Cheerios Milk & Cereal Bar	1 bar	2 exchanges
Chex Mix	1 bag	3 exchanges
Chocolate Milk	1 carton	2 exchanges
Chocolate Rice Krispie Treat	1 each	3 exchanges
Cracker Jacks	1 box	2 exchanges
Cranberry Juice	1 container (4 oz)	1 exchange
Flatbread Crackers	1 pkg	2 exchanges
Graham Crackers	1 package	1 exchange
Honey Wheat Braided Pretzels	1 bag	3 exchanges
Hot Chocolate	1 pkg	2 exchanges
Lorna Doones	1 package	2 exchanges
Mixed Nuts	¼ cup	3 exchanges
Nestles Crunch Granola Bar	1 package	2 exchanges
Orange	1 each	1 exchange
Orange Juice	1 container (4 oz)	1 exchange
Oreos	1 package	2 exchanges
Oyster Crackers	1 package	1 exchange
Peanut Butter	1 package	1 exchange
Pudding – all flavors	1 container	2 exchanges
Raisins	1 box	2 exchanges
Ritz Crackers	2 pkgs (4 crackers)	1 exchange
Skim Milk	1 carton	1 exchange
String Cheese	1 each	1 exchange
Teddy Grahams	1 package	1 exchange
Trail Mix Granola Bar	1 package	2 exchanges

Snack Time

Unlike meals, snack time at the EDC is held in the dayroom. At promptly 10:30 AM, 2:30 PM, and 8:30 PM, an RC comes out of the office, armed with meal cards and keys to the cupboards and the fridge. We are supposed to arrange ourselves in an orderly line, but more often than not we storm the cupboards in a frenzy of indecision.

"Should I get an apple or string cheese?"

It is never a question for me after I eat my first Cheerios bar. Prior to coming to the EDC, I had indulged in drinking maple syrup straight from the bottle, eating spoonful after spoonful of granulated sugar that I crunched gleefully between my molars because I loved the texture, and eating entire jars of jam (preferably strawberry). I also relished drinking half a bottle of soy sauce. I've had this flair for condiments since my preteen years. Brown sugar used to be a favorite, as were uncooked oats and the occasional chug of apple cider vinegar, straight from the bottle.

No one at the EDC will permit me to eat a jar of jam for snack or drink a bottle of soy sauce (and I am too mortified to ask), so instead I eat a Cheerios bar at every snack because it is the most sugar-filled food I can find at the EDC. Eventually my Cheerios bar consumption is outlawed, as staff thinks the bars are a "safe food" for me, meaning I am not "challenging" myself by trying different foods. They don't know I am simply enjoying a mini–sugar binge during snack time.

To make my Cheerios bar last, I dissect it. First, I separate the two layers that hold it together. Next, I eat the layer without icing. Then I pick the icing off the remaining layer, relishing the grit of sugar on my teeth. Last, I pluck at the denuded remainder of the bar.

While I am performing microscopic dissection on my Cheerios bar, Holly wolfs down her pretzels at lightning speed, then goes out on the deck for a postsnack cigarette, Danielle furtively stashes her Oreos in between the sofa cushions when she thinks no one is looking, and Sandra refuses to eat anything other than fruit because carbohydrates are "junk food." Laura eats her yogurt like a normal person and joins Holly on the deck, while Eliza is granted the privilege of choosing whether she wants to eat a snack, because she follows her meal plan and doesn't purge.

Occasionally, someone will flat-out refuse a snack or have a breakdown because no one has restocked the oyster crackers in the snack cupboard, and oyster crackers are their "safe food."

Even though we know the snack list by heart, we stare at it when we pass by. Food, our addiction and our fear, fascinates us. As much as we feign disinterest, we secretly all know the truth.

One day, at 1:30 PM, Holly attempts to break into the snack cupboard while yelling that she wants food—*now*. RC Allison tells her it is one thirty and she has to wait until snack time. Is Holly hungry?

We are always hungry.

DINING GUIDELINES

1. Residents are to follow the dining schedule.
2. All meals are to be eaten at the dining room tables.
3. All residents need to have their full meal at the table when being checked.
4. All residents must have their meal card checked during meals and snacks.
5. Conversations during meals should be encouraged to be not food related and or past eating disorder behaviors.
6. All residents must show their plate to the respective RC from their unit before emptying their plate. Residents will be marked as non compliant if they clear before showing staff their plate/bowls etc.
7. Residents are not allowed to rinse off any food in the dining room! NO EXCEPTIONS!!!!
8. Residents need to place dirty dishes in appropriate storage bins.
9. No dishes of any kind including cups, glasses and silverware may be taken from the dining room for any reason. Disposable dishes will be made available for staff who need to take food out of the dining room. *Disposable dishes may not be used by residents.*
10. Condiments will be available when the Dietitian's have determined them to be appropriate for the food that is being served at a specific meal. Residents are asked to take condiments to their table to add to food and not to open them or mix them with food at the counter.
11. Only one serving of vegetables per resident.
12. No caffeine allowed (unless it is provided by the Dietitian's for a challenge).
13. Residents may not be in the dining room without a staff member.
14. Residents may not leave the dining room without a staff member and the group.
15. Snacks must be eaten during the designated time on the schedule otherwise considered non-compliant.
16. Residents are not to refill Gatorade or any other bottles with drinking water. All bottles must be thrown out after use. All drink must be consumed in the dayroom or dining room. NO Food or Beverages allowed in the bedroom areas.
17. RCs have been instructed <u>to not call</u> down to the kitchen to receive items that have run out during a meal. The kitchen has been instructed to <u>not</u> bring up more side salad, vegetables, coffee, condiments etc etc.
18. Residents are responsible for getting their snack during the designated snack periods. RCs will not give a resident their snack after the designated snack period has expired.

Scenes from the Dining Room

OF THE EATING-DISORDERED

Elise is from Oregon, but there is something inherently
Californian about her—perhaps it's her dark tan and bleached
hair. Later, we find out that she lived in California and then
moved to Oregon to go to college. She is competition. Her
hip bones jut out and her arms look breakable. Elise has been
bulimic for a long time. During her first breakfast, she shocks
us by nonchalantly taking three (not one, but three) pieces
of bacon.

We watch her eat the bacon, then discuss it during our
postbreakfast cigarette (I'm not a smoker, but I occasionally filch
a cigarette). Laura is laying bets on when Elise will sneak down

the hall and purge; Danielle is too busy bouncing up and down on her tiptoes, trying to burn off the butter she put on her toast this morning. She says she can't remember what bacon tastes like. I haven't allowed myself to eat bacon in a long time.

During dinner I place two peas on my spoon and flick them in the direction of RC Evan. The peas whiz by him and bounce off the wall.

"Are you kidding me?" he says.

The whole table starts laughing.

Danielle is having a hard time finishing her Mexican tofu casserole. To distract her, I launch a cherry tomato at Sandra, who wipes off the tomato and eats it.

Danielle and Sandra jostle each other at the dining room door before every meal. As soon as the RC unlocks it, they sprint to the fruit basket. They are both in search of the coveted green apple. Sandra gets the apple, takes one bite out of it, and offers it to Danielle, who eats the whole thing, core included.

The fire alarm goes off in the middle of breakfast one morning in June and we shuffle outside, the bottoms of our pajama pants wet with dew. We shiver and smoke cigarettes until the all-clear signal is given and we can return to our food.

"Someone stole my toast!" exclaims Sandra.

"Some fuckstick probably binged on it," says Holly.

Eliza and I laugh as Sandra repeatedly voices her concern over her lack of toast, waving her skinny arms in the air, her voice edging on panic.

"Go ahead and get another piece and calm down," says RC Allison.

Sandra talks about her toast for the rest of the day, bringing it up in Group Therapy and during evening check-in. She twirls her hair with her index finger while recounting the story for the third time.

"No one cares about your motherfucking toast," Laura says in a calm voice.

Individual
Therapy

WITH THERAPIST ELAINE

I've had ten therapists, most of them ignorant about how to
treat eating disorders. Over the years I have been told I don't have
an eating disorder; it's perfectly normal for a teenage girl to diet;
I'm merely engaging in adolescent rebellion; this isn't serious; this
is a phase I will outgrow like last year's pants; if I wait fifteen minutes, the urge to purge will pass; I just need to make a meal plan; I
don't want to get better; this is all my parents' fault; I need to have
my chakras balanced; I need to learn the fine art of forgiveness; I'm
not thin enough for treatment, I'm not sick enough for treatment,
I'm obviously not trying hard enough to recover.

I have also been told I do have an eating disorder, this is not a normal teenage diet, this is more than adolescent rebellion, this is a serious illness, I'm slowly killing myself, I do want to get better, this is not anyone's fault, I need to stop numbing myself out and let myself feel anger without guilt, eating disorders are not about thinness, I need intensive treatment immediately.

At the EDC, Elaine is my therapist. She is our floor's Group Therapy leader and the person who conducts individual therapy sessions with each of us. Because I am so quiet at first, Elaine often forgets my name. Compared with the vocal bulimics and shockingly thin anorexics, I fade into the background, a silent observer, recording the scenes before me in my journal.

During our second session (our first session involved filling out the required paperwork), I tell Therapist Elaine about how I ended up at the EDC, about the events of the last year, about how desperate I was.

Therapist Elaine listens to this information with what I assume is an emotionless face. We play the therapy staring game. I know that I'm supposed to be crying, or at least showing some emotion, but I feel none. I am blank, and that is what I tell Elaine when she asks me how I feel. She tells me we will work on getting in touch with my emotions.

Emotions scare me. Emotions signal a loss of control, and I have tried so hard and for so long to be in control of as many things as possible in my life. Yet I sense that I am missing out on something, that my blank existence is no way to live. By engaging in eating-disordered activities, I am numbing my feelings.

Instead of feeling my anger, I throw it up; instead of feeling my sadness, I attempt to starve it away.

I've substituted school for intimacy, particularly as an undergraduate. Focusing on school to the extent that I did left me no time for intimate relationships, and that seemed like a good idea at the time, since the vulnerability an intimate relationship requires was something I sought to avoid.

As I sit here with Therapist Elaine, I'm dressed in pajama pants and a sweatshirt, with my blanket wrapped around me, and I begin to think that I am watching my life hurtle onward without me. I tell Elaine I want to work on my perfectionism, get in touch with my emotions, and learn how to live my life. And she tells me we will work on all of that.

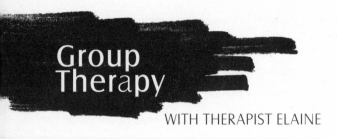

Group Therapy

WITH THERAPIST ELAINE

chairs and sofas in the day-
room

The chairs and sofas in the dayroom are arranged in a circle, to facilitate a feeling of closeness. The furniture is comfortable but worn and makes obscene noises when its occupants stand up. We fight over the lighting. Half of us like the dayroom dim and murky; it is easier to nap in the semilight of late afternoon. The other half want all the lights blazing and can't stand the gloom when the room is poorly lit.

Therapist Elaine sits in the therapist chair in front of the fireplace that we are not allowed to use. Whatever RCs are on duty sometimes sit in on Group Therapy and offer feedback. Therapist Elaine asks someone to start, and we go around the circle and talk about how we're doing today, what we're struggling with, and whether we need to take time to talk. We read assignments from Therapist Elaine that we have completed. This is called processing. At the end of Group Therapy, we all stand up and form a circle. Then we clasp hands and recite the Serenity Prayer.

There are perpetual sleepers in Group Therapy. Laura snuggles under her tie-dyed fleece blanket and curls up against whomever she is sitting on the sofa with. Danielle falls into such a deep sleep that she snores and has to be prodded awake. Those of us who aren't sleeping play Tetris or knit. Anything to occupy our hands. All of us have trouble sitting still. This time for contemplation makes us nervous.

Group Therapy is uneventful unless someone has a rape flashback or a breakdown brought on by the stress of telling the story of their trauma. We watch as other residents leave this reality and enter the past. Their eyes glaze over and they don't respond to anything, except when they jump or scream when touched. We watch, curled into ourselves, wrapped in blankets, as our peers relive trauma so unbearable that their minds overload. We grow educated about the signs of a flashback; we learn how to ground each other in the present.

Certain group members are prone to dramatic breakdowns. Sandra is known for bursting out of her seat in an explosion of bony limbs and wailing inconsolably. We question the authenticity of her episodes. She throws herself onto the floor, wiry arms sprawling in all directions. When Sandra has a breakdown,

Group Therapy ends because it is impossible to concentrate with her wailing in the background.

When Therapist Elaine goes on vacation in Siberia for two weeks, we get Arlene as a substitute therapist. We dub her Fuckstick Arlene because we like the sound of "fuckstick," a word that we believe we have created, and it seems to fit Arlene well. Fuckstick Arlene stares at us through large wire-frame glasses that emphasize her owlish appearance. She is a proponent of worksheets. We all fall asleep in Group Therapy, and after the first week most of us boycott it altogether because it has become Worksheet Therapy. In an effort to liven up Group Therapy and minimize the rate of attrition, Fuckstick Arlene announces that we will be going outside for Play Therapy. Intrigued, we follow her outside, where we find sidewalk chalk and balls. Fuckstick Arlene wants us to play Assertiveness Hopscotch, which involves stating a need every time you hop from square to square. None of us will play except for Laura, whose sarcasm goes undetected by Fuckstick Arlene. When Therapist Elaine returns from Siberia, I have to rein in the impulse to hug her and beg her to never leave us with Fuckstick Arlene again.

One afternoon in late June, Eliza and I are sitting on the coveted blue leather sofa during Group Therapy, wrapped in our blankets and watching as Laura comes down from a rape flashback, that glazed, faraway look in her eyes dissipating as she clenches an ice pack, concentrating on feeling the cold and staying present. Danielle is shaking her head back and forth, back and forth, her fluffy tufts of thin hair swaying methodically. Meanwhile, Sandra is gesturing wildly with her scrawny arms, telling Therapist Elaine and the rest of the group how she purged in a Tupperware container, wrapped it in paper, and gave it to her mother for Christmas.

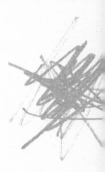

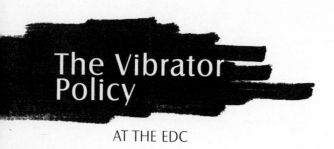

The Vibrator Policy

AT THE EDC

Before a Group Therapy session, we talk about how long it's
been since we had sex. Someone wonders whether we're allowed to
have vibrators. Sandra says she'll ask Therapist Elaine during Group
Therapy. None of us believe she will do it.

After checking in, Sandra says she has a question. Therapist
Elaine tells her to ask it.

"I was curious about what the vibrator policy is."

Silence. Therapist Elaine blushes. All the residents stare
at each other, then collapse into fits of immature giggles. This
is the most we've laughed in a long time. Our sides hurt and our
eyes tear up from laughing. We are all in our early twenties, but
we find this hilarious.

"I'm not sure. I don't think they're allowed, because it would violate your roommate's privacy. And we'd have to keep them in the office, in your personal bin, which means you would have to request to use them. Then, when you were done, you'd have to return them to the office, and that would be gross," says Therapist Elaine.

"Don't you want us to love our bodies and have positive sexual experiences?" asks Holly.

"Residential treatment is not the place for vibrators," says Therapist Elaine.

Confession

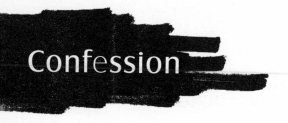

The first assignment Therapist Elaine gives me is to identify
my eating disorder behaviors and the negative consequences of
those behaviors. I sit in the conference room at the end of the hall
and listen to the Tori Amos *Little Earthquakes* CD as I complete
my first assignment. It takes me hours to compile my list of behaviors and consequences, and when I finish, I am appalled at how
long the list is. I know I will read it in Group Therapy the next
day, as that is what we do at the EDC—we all confess our sins
and then talk about how we feel. I've heard other people read their
lists and I am not nervous, as most everything has been mentioned
before. And so the next day, I read.

Therapeutic Exercise:

EATING DISORDER BEHAVIORS

Bingeing and purging

Purging after eating something with a high caloric or fat content

Taking diet pills with ephedrine even though I knew they were worsening my heart problems

Not getting dinner or drinks with friends after class because I couldn't deal with the food and eating in front of people

Not drinking alcohol because it has too many calories

Lying to friends about having eaten

Lying to friends about purging

Weighing myself multiple times a day

Restricting to only "safe" foods

Restricting my water intake

Running compulsively to burn calories or as punishment for bingeing

Fasting

Skipping meals

Not wearing a jacket when it was cold in an attempt to burn more calories

Spending hours in front of a full-length mirror, convinced I could actually see myself getting fatter

Obsessively fantasizing about liposuction

Bingeing and purging instead of dealing with what was upsetting me

Drinking large amounts of coffee and diet soda to mute my hunger and trick myself into feeling full

Counting out precise serving sizes

Eating one meal over the course of a day

Claiming I wasn't feeling well so I didn't have to eat

Avoiding friends so I could binge and purge

Only eating even numbers of things because odd numbers felt wrong

Therapeutic Exercise:

THE NEGATIVE CONSEQUENCES OF MY EATING DISORDER

(Physical Health Problems)

Heart problems (PVCs, PACs, and bradycardia)

Low and orthostatic blood pressure

Passing out and getting a concussion

Sore throat

Dizziness

Constipation

Bloating

Stomach pain

Headache

Electrolyte imbalances

Acid reflux

Cramping in extremities from low potassium

Weakened immune system

(Loss of Respect for Myself)

Lying to friends about eating disorder behavior

Too tired to go out

Feeling worthless because of my weight

Not having the energy to get out of bed

Neglecting my students' papers

Missing class

Pretending everything was okay even when it wasn't

*(How My Eating Disorder Has Affected
My Relationship with Others)*

Withdrew from friends and family

Having a short temper and no patience

Getting into arguments with friends about weight loss and
eating disorder behaviors

Losing several significant others because I was too wrapped up
in the eating disorder

Not wanting close friends because I didn't want to have to tell
them about the eating disorder

(Deterioration of Social Life Due to My Eating Disorder)

Isolating myself

Not answering my phone or returning messages

Distancing myself from friends

Not wanting to get to know people

Losing touch (on purpose) with friends

(School and Job Problems Due to My Eating Disorder)

Lack of concentration

Quitting my food service job because I didn't want to be around food

Missing class because I was ill or hospitalized

Cognitive problems because of my concussion

Skipping class because I was too tired to get out of bed

Having to wear a Holter Monitor to the last class I taught this past semester

Not being able to sit still during class because of all the caffeine and diet pills I consumed

(How My Eating Disorder Has Affected Me Spiritually)

I have become more isolated from people. I have a hard time trusting people, because I am afraid that if I tell them about the eating disorder, they will turn on me. Sometimes I get so caught up in the eating disorder that I don't see the world around me. My eating disorder has numbed me out. I am cut off from my essence. I feel like I have lost something vital to who I am, like I am a shell of the person I used to be.

(Loss of Control in Regard to My Eating Disorder)

My whole life feels out of control. I don't know when my body is going to fail me, like when I passed out. My purges increased when I tried to cut back. I kept setting goal weights, reaching them, and then going lower.

(*How I Hid My Eating Disorder from Others*)

I'd tell my friends I'd eaten, claim I was ill or not hungry. I'd avoid gatherings involving food. I'd purge in seldom-used bathrooms at school. I'd grocery shop at least half an hour from home. I'd fast before an event, so I could then allow myself to eat.

(*What I Have Lost*)

Not only have I lost weight, but I've also lost myself. I lost Diana, my ex-girlfriend, because I was emotionally numb and involved in my eating disorder. I've lost so much time that I could've spent doing something useful. I lost my confidence. I lost my will to live. I just went through the motions. I've lost academic opportunities. I've lost money. I've lost my health. I've lost my voice.

Everyone except Therapist Elaine stares out the window, because my list mimics everyone else's list. We have all lost, and sometimes given away, so much.

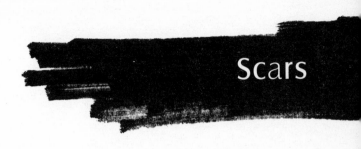

Scars

The scars on my body tell a story. The long, reddish weal on my left shin is where I scraped my leg on the pool ladder one summer. The shiny, raised bump on my chest is the result of scratching a chicken pox welt when I was seven. Under my chin, there is a raised line where I fell and hit the coffee table when I was learning to walk. My forehead bears an indented scar from my running into the same coffee table edge three times, hitting the exact same spot each time, while learning to walk.

Then there are the scars I carry inside my body: my eroded esophagus, corroded with stomach acid and bile; my heart that skips and flutters to an abnormal beat.

I am not the only one who carries such scars. One night when Holly lights up a cigarette, I see scar tissue on her inner arm. I glance at her arm and see FAT carved into her flesh. The scar is old and white against her tan skin. Laura took a razor to her abdomen; then the wounds got infected, and now she refuses to show anyone. Sandra hated herself so badly one night that she sliced horizontal cuts all the way from her wrist to her elbow. These cuts are not meant to kill, they are meant to create physical pain because physical pain is a distraction from mental anguish.

Holly's esophagus is riddled with tears and ulcers. Clots of blood erupt out of her mouth when she burps. Laura passes out when her heart rate becomes irregular. We are forever marked. Our bodies have borne witness to our madness, and they will never let us forget.

Autobiography

For my next assignment, Therapist Elaine asks me to write my autobiography and read it to the group in installments. Over the course of my first two months in treatment, I scrawl the details of my life in 130 notebook pages. I read each year in chronological segments during Group Therapy. There are parts I want to forget; there are parts I want to share.

Therapist Elaine, various RCs, and all the residents sit rapt in the dayroom and listen as I read the story of my life. I am our storyteller; perhaps something about my life resonates with my fellow residents as I read. By writing, I give my experiences a voice and I lend them credence, both for myself and for the others.

Some years were better than others. No matter how hard I try, I can't connect with what I read. Sometimes I cry when writing, but never when reading. This pattern worries my treatment team, and they keep telling me to let go, to let myself feel emotions as I read, but I don't know how.

I am not placing blame. I had a happy childhood spent running wild through the hills of rural Pennsylvania. I had Italian grandparents (my mother's parents) who doted on me and fulfilled my every whim. I had a proper British grandma, who talked in the soft speech of a woman raised outside London, and a Vietnam-haunted grandfather.

I had my own lavender bush that attracted fuzzy bees. I had parents who were high school sweethearts and too young to know better. I had Italian uncles and great-uncles who looked like gangsters and drank blackberry brandy in their coffee. Their laughter sounded like bells as they jostled me on their knees. I had a brother seven years younger than I whom I never understood.

My father and I tossed a football back and forth; my mother told me I could be anything I wanted to be when I grew up. My Italian grandparents sat with my mother and me during Mass on Sundays, then cooked a large spaghetti dinner, complete with portions for our dog. I drank tea with my British grandmother and listened to Michael Jackson and Cyndi Lauper with the bulky headphones she attached to the tape player. I grew up knowing I had possibilities and opportunities no one else in my family had. I grew up with the certainty that I would be one of the first people on either side of my blue-collar family to go to college.

I took dance lessons, gymnastics lessons, swimming lessons, French horn lessons, and flute lessons. I was baptized and confirmed in the Catholic Church. I had fish, dogs, and a cat. I had two parents who loved each other and never fought. I had all four grandparents alive and mostly healthy. I had neighborhood friends and trees to climb.

I am placing blame. I faced too much pressure to succeed and take advantage of the opportunities unavailable to previous generations of my family. I experienced the guilt and sexism of the Catholic Church. I was no good at math, no matter how hard I tried. Sometimes trying just wasn't good enough. I stopped dancing, swimming, and playing instruments. I refused to go to Mass. I did not fit the image of my family. I was the wild child, the intense, sensitive daughter whom my parents tried to rein in. I was explosive, depressed, and skeptical. I was not the daughter they thought I was.

RESIDENT OUTING GUIDELINES

1. On Sunday evenings, second shift RCs will help the group come up with an outing that week. Residents will complete the "Outing Request" form during check-in group on Sunday. An "outing" request folder will be provided on each floor/location. Residents may not sign up later than Sunday evening (unless they are away on pass). Residents should plan on attending the outing if they sign up. The Second Shift RCs will review the outing requests with the treatment team at a designated time that week. If no requests are given there will be no outing for that week or the RCs will pick an outing. Residents must be specific with the location and start and end time of the suggested outing. A back-up outing should be written as well.

2. The RC's and the Therapist will meet at 3:00 p.m. for a brief meeting to discuss the outing and passes for the weekend. The Therapist and second shift RCs will approve or not approve the outing. The RCs and treatment team members will decide together who will be eligible to attend the outing at that time.

3. Residents must be on YELLOW level to participate in the higher activity group outings (i.e. bowling, shopping etc.). Resident's on ORANGE Level may participate in low-level activities – per treatment team discretion (i.e. movie etc.). Residents, whose activity level changes the week of the outing, will be allowed to participate in the outing at the level they were at – per RC discretion. The following week they will be allowed to participate at their new level.

4. After the weekly "outing request" form has been completed, one of the RCs working should make one copy. The copy should go into the Charge Book. The original should be hung on the inside of the office window (facing out).

5. The RCs working Sunday evening are responsible for reserving a vehicle for that week's outing. The vehicle reserved and who reserved it should be noted on the outing request form and in the shift communication log.

6. On the night of the outing the RCs will make the decision based on staff available who will stay back with the residents and who will go on the outing. Acuity of the resident's left behind must be taken into consideration and if there are any safety concerns the RCs may cancel the outing. **Outings may be canceled for; inclimate weather, staffing issues, acuity issues, emotional concerns of residents or vehicle problems.** If more than 6 residents are going and two RCs need to go on the outing, one RC must call the Charge Person to let them know that both RCs will be going (This must be done before dinner). The floor going on the outing must also make prior arrangement for another floor to watch those residents that may stay behind. (Note: Two RCs <u>may only</u> go if more than 6 residents are participating in the outing).

7. The RCs may stop the outing and return to the Eating Disorder Center anytime during the outing if resident behavior / status is not safe (i.e. residents are purchasing/taking contraband, residents are not following directions from staff etc).

8. There will be <u>no</u> other stops made for any reason. Residents <u>may not be</u> dropped off for a pass. Staff may not stop at a convenience store/gas station to pick up cigarettes for residents. If the outing involves shopping, the group will be allowed 1 hour in the store.

9. All treatment guidelines set up for treatment applies for passes as well as outings. (i.e. no candy, gum, soda, caffeine unless otherwise specified. Residents are allowed one small popcorn, and one small non-diet caffeine free soda or drink at the movies)

10. Only **ONE** spontaneous "RC outing" on Saturday. RCs will choose the spontaneous outing from the following locations: Library, Barnes & Noble at Brookfield Sq., Blockbuster, Movie, Ben Franklin. Goodwill, Blockbuster (Belongings Run may only be done on a bi-weekly basis.). *Please see "RC Outing" guidelines for more information.*

11. Belongings run is separate from the weekly outing. Only residents that need to pick up supplies should be participating in the "belongings run". The "Belongings Run" is not to be used as a "shopping spree". The time should be used to pick up needed hygiene supplies (i.e. toothpaste, shampoo, etc.). Belongings Runs will occur on a bi-weekly basis. Belongings run can be done at Target, Kmart or Wal-Mart *(not Kohl's)*. *Please see "Belonging Run" guidelines for more information.*

12. Adolescent residents must remain with a staff member at all times while on an outing. Adult residents must remain with a buddy while on an outing and must be able to check in with staff. Residents are asked to empty their pockets and show their bags immediately upon returning from an outing or belongings run.

13. If the group decides to see a movie for their weekly outing. The movie that is to be seen needs to be written on the "outing suggestion form" (the treatment team needs to approve the appropriateness of the movie). Adolescent residents may not view rated "R" movies and adult residents may only view rated "R" movies with the approval of the treatment team. The group may not divide up and see different movies while at the movie theatre. The entire group must be seeing the same movie.

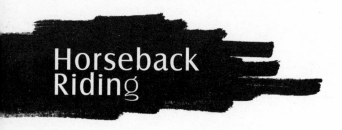

Horseback Riding

While we wait for Recreational Therapist Douglas to drive the van around to the front of the EDC, Laura braids my unruly hair into two French braids that hang just below my shoulders, and I don a black tank top and my least flattering pair of jeans. I am ready to go. Recreational Therapist Douglas herds Laura, Holly, Sarah, Courtney, Eliza, and me into the hospital van, and we're off to the farm.

In the van, Holly and I fight over the window seat, yelling at each other dramatically and bursting into laughter; Laura and Eliza fall asleep; and Courtney and Sarah sing along to the overplayed song "Roses" by OutKast that is once again playing on the radio.

Douglas just smiles to himself, after telling us that he is feeling particularly thankful that it is such a beautiful day and that he is sober (Douglas is in recovery from alcoholism).

At the stable, I am assigned a lazy chestnut roan who likes to snack on weeds alongside the trail. We aren't allowed to go any faster than a walk, but I press my thighs and knees into my horse and we begin to trot. Immediately, Recreational Therapist Douglas demands that I stop. Frustrated, I remember riding bareback in upstate New York on the biodynamic, organic farm where I worked a few summers ago, and riding a friend's horse on the dirt roads of northern Pennsylvania.

All I want is to gallop, to feel the wind whip my braids about my face and feel the horse's muscles ripple beneath my thighs. Instead, my horse meanders sedately along the trail while I listen to the other women talk about how exciting this foray into the countryside is. Laura and I exchange looks and roll our eyes at those city girls.

When we get back to the EDC, I smell like horse and feel fat in my unflattering jeans (they accentuate the wideness of my hips). We arrive in time for a pre-lunch Group Therapy session, during which I talk about feeling trapped in my body and trapped in my life; there are certain things I want to do, and there are things I need to do, and there are cultural and familial expectations to deal with, and all of these make me panic because there are too many expectations and I know I can't meet them and I just want everyone to leave me alone.

Laura says she can relate. Everyone in her family wants her to become an orthodontist and become her father's partner in his orthodontic practice. She wants to be a forensic scientist and study serial killers.

Everyone else sits around, staring off into space.

I feel better for getting this issue out in the open. Laura and I bond over our supposedly perfect families. We are the flawed daughters who need to be hidden away. We are the crazy Berthas secluded in the attic. My parents don't tell anyone where I am, except for one set of grandparents, my brother, one aunt, and one uncle. I am a secret burden, I have fucked up undeniably, and my parents are ashamed of me and horrified that their daughter has an eating disorder.

They claim this isn't so—they just don't want to broadcast private information in a public way, and if they tell the rest of my family, then word will leak out and the entire town will know, and my parents just want everybody to stay out of their business. We do live in a small town (population: 950 and shrinking), and word does get around.

I invite my parents to Family Weekend at the EDC, so they can meet with the parents of the women on my floor, and attend lectures about dealing with and supporting someone recovering from an eating disorder. Family Weekend coincides with my cousin's graduation party, and since my parents can't miss the graduation party without having a good explanation, they tell me they can't come.

In my mind, Family Weekend is more important than a graduation party. Once again, my parents' need for everything to appear perfect comes before my needs. I spend several Group Therapy sessions talking about how angry with and disappointed in my parents I am. We argue over the phone. Finally, they agree to come to the EDC another weekend. I'd like my parents to acknowledge that I am asking for help, and that I need them, and to not make me feel like I am an inconvenience.

Psychodrama

We are doing a psychodrama about family secrets, and Rachel has picked me to be the protagonist. Prior to the psychodrama, I was in a good mood. It is Tuesday, and we're going roller skating after dinner tonight. In preparation for this venture into the real world, I have put on jeans and a fitted purple shirt and done my makeup. My hair cascades over my shoulders and I tuck it behind my ears. Looking in the mirror, I realize the dark circles are gone from under my eyes and my skin has a glow. My body is slowly recovering.

"I want you to arrange the furniture in this room to resemble the setup of your living room in Pennsylvania," says Rachel.

I move three chairs together to represent a sofa and two chairs together to represent a love seat, and leave one chair out to represent an ottoman. I pull a blue mat in front of the simulated sofa to represent a fireplace. The other residents are sitting in chairs or on the floor. I cross my arms over my chest as my cheeks flush with nervousness.

"Pick someone to represent your mother, your father, and your brother," says Rachel.

I pick three residents and arrange them in my pseudo–living room. Mom and Dad sit together on the sofa, and my brother sprawls on the love seat. I occupy the ottoman chair.

"Are your parents happy together?" asks Rachel.

"Yes, I've only seen them fight once in my life."

"What about your brother?"

"He's sixteen and at a boarding school in northern Ohio. We're not close; he's seven years younger than me."

"Say something to your mother," says Rachel.

"I'm never good enough for you," I say.

"Switch places with your mother and sit beside Dad on the sofa. How would your mother respond to what you just said?"

"Nicole is immature. She exaggerates. Her father and I push her because she has so many opportunities we never had. She's a smart girl, but she doesn't work up to her potential. She puts a lot of pressure on herself and blames it on us," I say.

"How does that make you feel, Nicole? What do you want to say back to your mom?"

"I know you and Dad only want the best for me, but you push me so hard that I feel like nothing is ever good enough. You didn't go to college, but that was your choice."

"Nicole, I want you to tell us one of the secrets of your family," says Rachel.

I sit on the ottoman, legs crossed, staring at the wall. I don't want to do this. I want dinner to be over with and I want to fly around the roller-skating rink, arms outstretched in a flurry of speed.

"I have an eating disorder."

I'm shaking and my anger is rising.

"You've been angry lately; would you like to hit something?"

"Yes."

Rachel retrieves a Wiffle Ball bat and drags the cube-shaped blue mat to the center of the room. I've seen other residents do this, and I am ready.

"I want you to hit the mat as hard as you can and scream why you are angry at your parents."

At first I just beat the hell out of the mat because I can't verbalize. Then I start swinging and screaming. The litany of my anger goes like this:

"I'm angry that I'm never good enough for you."

"I'm angry that you didn't believe that I had an eating disorder."

"I'm angry that you don't listen to me."

"I'm angry that you live vicariously through me."

"I'm angry that you won't let me tell people where I am."

"I hear you have some perfectionist tendencies, Nicole. You have perfect posture when you swing the bat—were you a dancer?"

"Yes."

"You don't have to be perfect, Nicole. Pick someone to represent your eating disorder."

"Holly."

"Holly, put your arm around Nicole's neck. Nicole, keep yelling things and hitting the mat."

Now I'm heaving Holly's weight and my own, and I can't swing as well as I want to, and that irritates me.

"I'm angry that I couldn't trust you."

"I'm angry that you didn't offer to help me pay for treatment."

"Holly, I want you to tighten your arm around Nicole's neck."

I can't breathe and I panic, choking out, "Rachel, I . . . can't . . . breathe." Holly starts to relax her grip as she hears the panic in my voice, but Rachel tells her to tighten it back up. Tears form in the corners of my eyes and I can feel blood pounding in my head. Holly and I stand there, locked together.

"Why don't you fight back, Nicole?"

With all my might, I wrest myself free from Holly's grip and gulp air. I know Rachel is trying to evoke feeling in me, but other than my panic about being choked and my receding anger at my parents, I am numb.

"Are there any people in your life who love you unconditionally and accept you for who you are?"

"My maternal grandparents."

"Pick two people to represent them, and sit between them."

My parents won't let me tell my grandparents I am in treatment, because they think my grandparents won't understand. My grandparents think I'm temping in Minneapolis. I haven't called them for over a month, and I miss them so badly that I can't hold back the tears. My grandparents rub my back and tell me I'm beautiful and they love me no matter what. This knowledge makes me miss them more because, pretend as I might, I can't transform the two anorexics beside me into my lovely Italian grandparents.

Geriatric Skate

After dinner, RC Julia brings Big Red

After dinner, RC Julia brings Big Red (the hospital van) around
front and we pile in and head for the local Skateway Roller Rink. I
am trying to hang on to my post-psychodrama grumpiness, but it is
hard to do so when everyone is singing along to "Dirrty," by Christina
Aguilera, and gyrating in their seats. The only one of us who can sing
is Eliza, who is a voice major at a private college in the Twin Cities.

At Skateway we jump out of the van and make RC Julia take
pictures of us. We do this on all our outings; we feel the need to
record our time in treatment as a testament to our experiences.
After we pose for pictures, we enter Skateway and pay $3 to rent
ancient skates that squeak as we roll onto the wooden floor. I am

wishing that I'd brought my Rollerblades with me, but I didn't think treatment would incorporate roller skating.

Holly immediately starts racing around the rink in an effort to burn calories. Eliza and I hold hands and skate, and Holly flies by, shouting, "Lesbians!" We catch up to her and grab her hands, laughing as she tries to break free. RC Julia sits on the side with the residents who are not medically stable enough to roller-skate.

Courtney and Sarah skate backward, and I'm the first to wipe out.

Then, in come six elderly couples. The men are dressed in their Sunday best, and the women sport neon spandex costumes, complete with tights. We all glance at each other, wondering what parallel universe we have just entered. The music in the rink suddenly changes to a polka, and the couples begin partner skating. They take over the rink.

All of us huddle around RC Julia, whispering about this geriatric coup d'état. One of the couples skates over to us and informs us that we have infringed on Couples' Night. Apparently, the couples are part of a skating club, and this is their practice time. The only way we can skate is if we skate as couples. We agree to try it.

An elderly man in a cowboy hat asks Holly if he can have this skate. Holly's eyes widen, but she agrees.

A wizened man with arthritic fingers asks if I will skate with him. I say yes.

We skate side by side, his gnarled fingers gripping my forearm tightly. His name is Dale. He asks me if I'm from around here, and I panic. I don't want to tell Dale that we are EDC patients. The words come out of my mouth before I think.

"Oh, we're just sorority sisters from the University of Minnesota. We're having a reunion and we figured skating sounded like fun," I say.

"Well, isn't that something?" says Dale.

He proceeds to tell me about his grandchildren, and how he is a graduate of the University of Wisconsin. I glance over at RC Julia, who is having a hard time keeping a straight face. She pulls out my camera and begins snapping pictures. I notice Dale's blue-haired skating partner sulking in the shadows.

"Is that your wife?"

"Sure is."

"You should skate with her."

"Okay. Thanks for the dance."

"Oh no, thank *you*."

I skate over to RC Julia. Everyone has their skates off and their shoes on.

"Are you ready to go? Or do we need to give you a few minutes alone with your new boyfriend?" Holly asks.

"Miss Nicole, I can't believe you actually skated with him," says RC Julia.

"Holly did it too," I say.

"Yeah, but you liked it," says Holly.

We talk about Geriatric Skate for the rest of the summer. Whenever an RC asks us where we want to go, we always say Skateway, but only if it's Geriatric Skate.

Parents' Visit

y parents arrive at the edc at night My parents arrive at the EDC at night, via rental car, after flying

into the Milwaukee airport earlier in the day. I am sitting out front

with Holly, waiting for them to pull up, when they call my cell

phone. They are lost on the hospital grounds and have ended up on

an access road. I'm trying to give my mother directions, despite not

knowing exactly where she is, and I can hear the tension in her voice

over the static of our poor connection.

They pull into the EDC lot in a red car with Iowa plates, and

I think about how I've never been to Iowa. As my parents get out

of the car, I can see that their outfits are color-coordinated. They

always say they don't plan it, but as I grow older I am beginning to wonder. These are the people who joke that they bought our yellow Labrador retriever, Katie, because she matched their living room carpet.

We hug and I can tell they are nervous. I'm nervous too. I am not the daughter they thought I was. I spent an hour before the bathroom mirror, trying to tame my curly hair and get my makeup just right. Every outfit I tried on made me feel fat. Finally, I settled on my favorite jeans and a red short-sleeved shirt.

I introduce them to Holly and we head inside. I show them the dayroom, where Laura and Eliza are making a fleece blanket. My mother asks to use the bathroom and is surprised that there is no lock on the door. I show them the room I share with Laura, and they say how nice it is.

They have brought me a new cell phone, a pair of black pajama pants, and a white tank top, both of which are too small. I give them to Laura.

My mother chats with RC Marie, marveling at her Wisconsin accent, while my dad and I sign the pass forms so my parents can take me off the hospital grounds. Once we are in the car, we decide to go to Pepino's, an Italian restaurant in town. This is the first time I will eat with my parents since I told them about my eating disorder (I called them three weeks before I checked myself into the EDC). They order French silk pie and I order coffee. I savor it, dumping three packets of Equal into it. My mother tells me I won't sleep tonight, but the luxury of coffee takes precedence over sleep. When the pie comes, I take one bite and leave the rest to my parents.

We talk about my grandparents, my brother, and what is going on in our hometown. We don't talk about the fact that I'm EDNOS or that I'm in treatment. Therapist Elaine has advised both parties to keep the conversation light and just enjoy each other's company this weekend.

After an hour of innocuous conversation, it's time to head back to the EDC. My parents hug me and tell me goodnight, and that they'll see me after breakfast the next morning. When I get back to the EDC, RC Caroline asks me how it went and I tell her it was fine.

On Saturday morning I call my parents after breakfast. They pick me up at the EDC, but before we leave I show them the Art Therapy room. Its walls are covered in residents' artwork, mainly life-size outlines of how they perceive their bodies. My parents grow silent as they walk around the quiet room, witnessing the distorted vision and self-hatred of the eating-disordered. They don't stay long; it's a hard and somber place. None of my artwork is hanging on the walls; I have not gotten that far in Art Therapy yet.

We decide to drive to Old World Wisconsin, a tourist attraction that depicts life in a nineteenth-century Scandinavian settlement in Wisconsin. It is a bright Midwestern day, and my parents and I walk from village to village, inspecting farmhouses and learning how to card wool. I worry that I am losing weight from all the walking, and that I will get in trouble with Dietitian Caroline.

We eat lunch in the Old World Wisconsin cafeteria, where I realize I will never be able to accommodate my meal plan. I order a grilled chicken breast on a bun and a snack-size bag of chips. Compared with my parents, I eat slowly, and I can't finish my sandwich.

My dad and I wait outside the cafeteria while my mother uses the restroom. He tells me I have something hanging out of my nose, and I tell him it is my nose ring. I can tell he is burning to make a comment about it, but he doesn't. That would break the easygoing tone of the weekend.

We spend the rest of the day driving around rural Wisconsin, and my dad keeps saying it looks just like Pennsylvania. At some point I fall asleep in the back seat, like I did when I was little. I am exhausted from my foray into the outside world, and from trying to keep the peace with my parents.

Later, we stop at Target, where I pick up a few necessities, and then they drop me off in time for dinner at the EDC. At some point after waking up from my nap in the back seat, I've grown anxious and nervous. Back at the EDC, I eat dinner as fast as possible and sit on the deck with the other residents. I bum a smoke off Holly, and my hands shake with anxiety and the desire to purge. When RC Caroline tells us we are going to the movies, I immediately begin plotting how I will sneak away from the other women and purge.

The van ride to the cinema is nerve-racking. I tune out the conversation around me and instead obsess about how many calories I have already digested. At the cinema, my chance to purge comes when Eliza wants to get a drink. While we wait in line at the concession stand, I say I have to use the restroom.

I walk into a stall and purge my dinner. When I come out, Eliza is none the wiser. After the movie I see my parents walking out, and that adds to my stress.

That night, I talk to RC Caroline and Cindy about purging, and RC Caroline has me write a Reasons Not to Purge List.

Reasons Not to Purge
- My heart problems.
- Electrolyte levels.
- Orthostatic blood pressure.
- It's not going to get rid of the feelings or the pain.
- It's not going to make me feel better.
- It won't make me thin, and thin won't make me happy.
- I'm going to regret doing it.
- I'm going to feel terrible physically and emotionally.
- I want to enjoy my life, not spend it with my head over the toilet.
- I don't want to die.

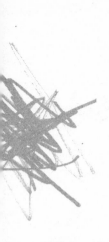

My parents fly back to Pennsylvania, and I can breathe again. But something has happened. They have triggered a reaction, an emotional response, within me, something I don't understand.

Transformations

er my parents visit i cut
f one foot of my hair

After my parents' visit, I cut off one foot of my hair. It is not premeditated. Eliza decides to shave her head, and as Laura runs the razor over Eliza's scalp (with staff permission), Eliza begins to weep. Clumps of ash-blond dreadlocks fall to the floor.

I tell Eliza I will cut my hair, too, in solidarity. I pull my thick, curly hair into a ponytail, then braid it. In the staff office, I request a pair of scissors and play with the end of the braid as I walk down the hall.

The scissors are dull. Laura saws through my thick braid and then trims up the ends. My hair rests just above my chin when she finishes. Everyone exclaims, "I like it!" and I shake my head from side to side. It feels so light. Laura jokes that I have just lost five pounds.

I walk into the staff office, and Marie and Evan, the two RCs on duty, say they like it because they can see my face now. I had so much hair before. They run their hands over Eliza's shiny head.

The next morning I realize I can no longer hide behind my hair, and I think short hair makes me look fat. Now my neck, shoulders, and upper arms are exposed. I hadn't realized how attached I was to my hair, or how much a part of my identity it was.

I think back to when I shaved my head in high school. I spent my junior and senior years at a boarding school hidden among the Tuscarora Mountains, on the Pennsylvania/Maryland border. When I started there, my hair was just below my shoulders. One day, I stood in front of the mirror in the communal girls' bathroom and hacked angrily into my hair with a pair of scissors. My best friend, Jane, watched in amazement as chunks of it landed on the tile floor.

A few weeks later, I decided to shave my head. I borrowed a pair of clippers from a faculty member and had another student run them over my head until nothing was left but a fine, dark stubble. Most of the girls who gathered in the bathroom to witness this transformation were not my friends. They came to watch out of pure curiosity. They gazed, wide-eyed and shocked, while they ran their manicured fingers through their own thick locks. A few rubbed my smooth head in admiration.

Looking in the mirror now, I see how different I look. People can see my face. I can't hide behind a curtain of curly hair any longer. Part of me misses all that hair that separated me from the rest of the world. But a weight has been lifted from me, and I am so much lighter now.

Some of Us Are Just Passing Through

Elise left the EDC early because her insurance refused to pay for treatment, despite the fact that she was thirty pounds underweight and had osteoporosis at age nineteen. Candace signed herself out AMA (against medical advice) when she panicked over her weight gain. Melanie's parents had enough money to pay for only one month of treatment, even though she needed at least two. Cynthia was asked to leave when she came back from pass drunk. While there is a core group of us throughout the summer, other residents pass through, sometimes before we learn their names. They leave pieces of themselves behind—an Art Therapy collage, an incomplete Group Therapy assignment—as the summer stretches on, but those who just pass through are not forgotten.

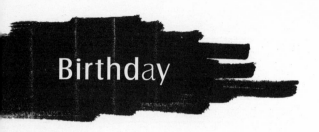

Birthday

ppy birthday princess "Happy birthday, princess," Holly shouts as she jumps on me, and we both fall onto the sofa in the dayroom. Laura produces a red construction-paper birthday crown and places it on my head. I start to pull my hair back into a ponytail, forgetting momentarily that I don't have long hair anymore. Eliza gives me a hug, and I run my hand over her newly shaved head for good luck. Sarah, Courtney, Danielle, and Sandra hug me and slip me a small envelope. I open it to find a $25 gift certificate from Barnes & Noble. I fight back tears as I thank everyone. I wasn't expecting this.

"It's time to feed the eating-disordered," Holly shouts. RC

Evan and RC Allison unlock the door to the dining room, and we shuffle in for breakfast. On the wall is a banner reading HAPPY BIRTHDAY, NICOLE, and all the residents on First Floor have signed it. Laura starts singing "Happy Birthday," and I flush a brilliant shade of scarlet and call her a fuckstick as I sit down with my plate.

"So, you still want to go ice skating in Milwaukee for our outing, right?" asks Holly. I've been allowed to pick where we go for our weekly outing, since it's my birthday.

"Yeah, and then I want to go to Caribou Coffee and get *caffeinated* coffee for a snack challenge. I think I almost have Dietitian Caroline convinced that it's a good idea."

"If anyone is going to convince Dietitian Caroline to let us get caffeine, it's going to be you. She thinks you're mature and a good influence on everyone," says Sarah.

"That's because she leaves at 5:00 PM and I don't get crazy until after dinner," I say.

We finish our breakfast and move to the deck, where Courtney gives me a cherry-flavored cigarette. After I'm done smoking it, I continue to periodically lick the filter, since it tastes of sugar. I inch over to the patio door and look at my reflection in the full-length glass. All of the mirrors in the EDC are tiny and nailed high up on the wall so that we cannot scrutinize our bodies. However, the staff does not realize that the patio door is essentially a full-length mirror. After glancing at my reflection, I decide that my current outfit of pajama pants and a sweatshirt makes me look fat, so I go to my room and search through my drawers for something more flattering.

I decide on jeans and a fitted red T-shirt. Then I decide that the T-shirt is too fitted; I don't want anyone to see my figure today. I find a shirt that snaps up the front, but that makes me look like I have more love handles than I actually do. Maybe pajama pants and a sweatshirt are the way to go. At this point, I have clothes strewn all over the floor. Laura comes in, looks at me, looks at the pile of clothes, and propels me out the door.

"You are not changing your outfit any more today," she says.

"But I look fat."

"No, you don't."

RC Allison comes out of the office and looks at me suspiciously. She has caught on to my habits.

"Were you in there changing clothes?" she asks.

"Yes."

"Well, no more—don't give in to your eating disorder."

I head to the dayroom, where I sulk through Group Therapy. I perk up when Dietitian Caroline announces that we will be allowed to order caffeinated coffee at Caribou Coffee after we go ice skating tonight. But we're still not allowed to use artificial sweeteners or skim milk.

The rest of the day flies by in a whirlwind of therapy. Right before dinner, I decide I cannot wear pajama pants and a sweatshirt to go out. I start trying on clothes, throwing them all around the room as anger builds within me. My clothes don't fit right anymore;

I've gained weight and I want to cry and scream with frustration and anger. Eliza comes in and drags me out of the room. RC Evan is standing in the hall.

"How many times have you changed clothes today?" he asks.

"Thirteen."

"Do not let your body image sabotage your night out," he says.

After dinner, RC Julia tells us she is not driving Big Red to Milwaukee, which means no ice skating. Instead, we go mini-golfing. I hate mini-golf; I always swing too hard and get frustrated because I never win. Still, I agree to give it a try. Besides, we will still be getting caffeinated coffee, and that's going to be the high point of the night, anyway.

In the van, I get the coveted shotgun seat, as well as control of the radio, which I tune to classic rock, amid groans from the other residents. RC Julia and I talk as she drives. Whenever RC Caroline or RC Julia drives us anywhere, I always vie for shotgun so I can talk to them. They talk about topics other than eating disorders. One day I convinced RC Caroline to give us the scenic tour of the local town, partly because I didn't want to go back to the EDC, and partly because I wanted to talk to her about her former job as a social worker for Planned Parenthood. When I sit shotgun with RC Julia driving, we talk about her upcoming marriage and my experiences in graduate school.

At the mini-golf course, our group's dysfunction level soars. Laura mutters and swears when she hits the ball into a water hazard, Holly throws her club into the air like a baton, Courtney and Sarah grow aloof, and Eliza tries to persuade everyone to get along. I, predictably, hit the ball onto I-94 in a fit of anger. After the eighth hole, we ask RC Julia if we can quit and just go get coffee. She thinks that's a good idea.

On the way to Caribou Coffee, Holly leans in behind RC Julia and sticks her lit lighter in her face while Julia is trying to make a left turn. I know this is dangerous, but I can't help but laugh. At the coffee shop, we pile out of the van and fight each other to be the first person in line for coffee. All of us order medium Caramel Coolers, and when RC Julia isn't looking, we ask for extra shots of espresso.

We sit on the patio, watching the sun melt below the horizon. RC Julia says we all look so happy, and she takes a picture of all of us with my camera. Then Laura and Holly lean in and kiss each of my cheeks, and even though Julia thinks the gesture is inappropriate, she takes a picture anyway. When I get this roll of film developed, I don't recognize myself, with my hair hovering above my chin and my eyes looking off to the side in uncharacteristic shyness. And, I wonder, when did I grow so unsure of myself?

Holly gives me a piggyback ride to Big Red, and Sarah takes a picture of our butts. We are all caffeinated and giddy on the way back to the EDC. Then, halfway through the ride, we crash, and everyone falls asleep except RC Julia and me. I stare out the window, watching the grass and trees roll by in a smear of green.

"What are you thinking about, Miss Nicole?" asks RC Julia.

"My other birthdays. For the past two years I've had ridiculously large parties with lots of alcohol, and now I'm happy with caffeinated coffee."

"Well, just think about how much more fun your birthday will be next year, when you're healthy," says RC Julia.

I look over at her and smile.

"I know you're going to beat this, Nicole," says RC Julia.

I think this is the best part of my birthday. RC Julia believes in me.

Desperation

e are desperate.
r eating disorders are
addiction, and we want to
ccumb to them.

We are desperate. Our eating disorders are an addiction, and we want to succumb to them. We try to engage in eating disorder behavior whenever we think no one is looking, or we do it blatantly until we are told to stop. Danielle tends to hide in her closet. Rather than admitting that she is exercising in there, she claims she is masturbating. Courtney sneaks out the front door and goes running in the woods. She comes back sweaty and claims that it's just hot outside. Laura stashes her nuts down her pants at dinner, then dumps them in the toilet. I habitually sneak down the hall when no one is looking (or when I think no one is looking) and ram my fingers down my throat and purge my meals. When I hear the *clomp* of RC Julia's boots against the floor, the sound coming closer to the bathroom, I panic and attempt to finish my purge before she swings open the bathroom door and finds me slumped over the toilet, hand coated in mucus and food chunks, tears streaming down my face.

Not until years later will I realize just how desperate most of us were, shaking our legs to burn calories, going on secret missions to purge, and telling never-ending lies to cover up our eating disorder behavior. At the time, all of those actions were part of everyday life; to us they had become normal.

Monday 11/18
1 english muffin - 130 cals
1 tsp butter - 50 cals
1 english muffin - 130 cals
1 tsp sugarfree jelly - 25 cals
1 banana - 100 cals
1/2 cup special K - 100 cals
1/2 cup nonfat skim - 50 cals
1 packet nonfat low cal hotchocolate - 25 cal
1 cup skim - 50 cals
1 g sugar free jello - 10 cals
= 680 calories

Tuesday 11/19 - 141 lbs
- 1 english muffin - 130 cals
- 1 tsp butter - 50 cals
- 1 cup nonfat yogurt - 100 cals
- 2 granola bars - 180
- 1 creamer - 20 cals
- 1 cup skim - 50 cals
- 2 slices fat free bread - 160
- 2 slices tofu cheese - 80 cals
- 1 small can tuna - 80 cals
- 1 sugar free jello - 10 cals   = 860 calories

wednesday
- cup apple cider - 90 cals
- 1 can veggie soup - 180 cals
- 1 salt free rice cake - 35 cals
- 1 tsp jam - 50 cals
- 1 cup special k - 100 cals

- 1/2 cup nonfat slim - 50 cals
- 1 sugar free jello - 10 cals
- 1 grapefruit - 39 cals

354 cals

Thursday - 143 lbs
- nofat yogurt 100 cals
- 2 granola bars - 180
- 1 can soup - 180
- 1 rice cake - 35
- 1 tsp jam 50 cals
- 1 grapefruit - 39 cals
- 1 glass ultra slim - 90 cals
- 1 diet hot chocolate - 25 cals

= 699 cals

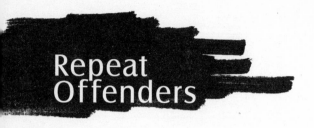

Repeat Offenders

Holly has been to the EDC twice before; Danielle has been
three times. Repeat offenders are common. It's easy to end up back
at the EDC: It's safe and predictable, you are taken care of, and you
have someone to talk to at all hours of the day and night. It's easy
to run scared from health and life, and to slip back into sickness.
Most residents don't achieve health and recovery on the first try, and
repeat offenders are more common than you would think. Throughout the summer, I try to decide if I want to be a repeat offender, but
I can't come to a conclusion.

Heart Trouble

I've just turned twenty-three, and I've been at the EDC for a month. Holly is curled up beside me on the blue leather sofa in the dayroom, right before Art Therapy. My arms hug my knees to my chest, and I am trying to stay calm and breathe. Is this a panic attack or a heart attack? My heart is pounding so hard, I think it's liable to thump its way out of my chest. I picture my damaged heart lying bloody at my feet. The beat is so erratic that Holly can't take my pulse.

In the RC office, my heart rate is 105 (my baseline is 40) and my blood pressure is registering at 130/110, compared with my baseline of 86/58. Now there is a throbbing pain in my chest and it hurts to inhale. Shannon and Brett, the two RCs on duty, page the health supervisor, who sends me to the emergency room. This is my sixth emergency room visit in two years for heart trouble.

At the hospital, I'm hooked up to an EKG that registers premature atrial contractions, premature ventricular contractions, and abnormal sinus pauses. My potassium levels are low again, which affects the rhythm of my heart. I am given IV fluids and potassium, then released.

If I continue to engage in eating disorder behavior, I will be in danger of further heart damage and a heart attack. But two days after my emergency room visit, my head is back over the toilet. I slip down the hall after dinner, when the RCs are busy giving everyone their after-dinner Maalox and Tums. I take off my shoes so no one will hear me glide down the hall, and I shut the bathroom door cautiously, taking care not to make noise. Then I quietly heave up the contents of my stomach until nothing but acid comes up. I lay my head against the toilet seat, relieved that I am empty again.

Nutrition Group

NORMAL EATING IS

eating when you're hungry

and stopping when you're full.

It's eating healthy foods,

but treating yourself occasionally.

ormal eating is

it's eating healthy foods.
but treating yourself occasionally

Johannsonator
Sessions

august johannson is my psychiatrist

Dr. August Johannson is my psychiatrist while I am at the EDC.
When we are not in his presence, we call him the Johannsonator,
or Augie. He is a quiet and thoughtful man, an ex–lacrosse player
for the University of Wisconsin, who walks with a swagger and has
a shy Midwestern smile. Several residents have intense crushes on
him. Whenever his back is turned, Courtney does hip thrusts and
makes an orgasm face behind his back, which sends us into gales of
giggles. The consensus on the floor is that most everyone would fuck
the Johannsonator if given the chance (I, however, would not). I tend
to think this sexual fascination with him comes from the power he
holds over us. He decides if we get solo walks (the privilege of walk-

ing around the hospital grounds unsupervised) and what medications we are given, and, most important, he is the one who decides when we are well enough to discharge.

During my time at the EDC, I am not on any psychiatric meds, although I spend many of my Johannsonator sessions begging for Ativan or Xanax because I'm having massive anxiety attacks that leave me curled in a ball on the sofa, feeling like I'm dying of that heart attack I used to wish for. The Johannsonator thinks I need to experience my feelings instead of numbing them out with eating disorder behavior or medication; therefore, he will not prescribe me anything but Prozac, which I refuse to take because of a horrible experience I had with Paxil when I was seventeen. (I had withdrawal when I stopped taking it, even though I tapered the dosage as my doctor directed me to.)

Because we don't have much to talk about in the way of medication, the Johannsonator and I talk about my body image (it's usually atrocious). He asks me about my body image and I start crying, and he says, "I'm guessing this means it's not too good." Then we argue about whether my weight is stable (I say no, he says yes), and then we are done until the next week, when we have the same conversation again.

However, sometimes we also talk about my parents, and how they think everything I do is meant to get their attention or to rebel against them. For example, I pierced my nose and they thought it was a direct attack on their values. I pierced my nose because I find nose rings aesthetically pleasing. My parents sometimes forget that

I am no longer an angry adolescent determined to get a rise out of them. I respect the Johannsonator because, unlike other medical professionals I have dealt with, he does not talk to me in a condescending manner. He sees me as an individual, not as a disorder, which is refreshing, as some of the staff members at the EDC are prone to lumping all of the residents into a homogenous eating-disordered group.

The Johannsonator and I discuss what my main issues are, and we agree that I struggle with perfectionism academically and in relation to my body. I internalize my emotions and put up a strong front until I explode in a ball of rage or eating disorder behavior. (My symptoms tend to follow a cycle: It worsens during the school year and it starts as restricting myself.) When Rachel, the psychodrama counselor, questions the degree to which I drank during college, the Johannsonator understands when I tell him I am not an alcoholic, although I admit to having abused alcohol in college, like so many other college students.

In an atmosphere that can be best described as chaotic, my weekly Johannsonator sessions keep me grounded. They are part of how I learn to trust people again, and to open up.

Art Therapy

t therapy stresses me out Art Therapy stresses me out. I am expected to express emotions I cannot verbalize; I am supposed to leave the realm of words. These prospects terrify me, and in protest, all my paintings (I refuse to do anything other than paint) have words on them. There is a series of projects to work on in Art Therapy, including the History Behind Your Eating Disorder project, the Body Perception project, Half Trace/Half Perception, Full Body Trace, and the Discharge Anxiety project.

Art Therapist Tracy picks what she thinks is an appropriate project for me.

The Half Trace/Half Perception project makes me hate my

body with an unprecedented level of intensity.
For this project, I cut a sheet of paper taller than
I am and paint it orange with swirls of white
and red. Next, I draw a line down the center of
the paper. On one half of the paper I draw how
I perceive my body (just the left side). Tracy
has me lay the paper flat on the ground, and she
traces my right side, so that half of the paper is
my perceived body image, and the other half is
my actual body outline.

My perception is completely out of
proportion with my actual body. In my distorted vision my arms are thicker, my waist
less defined, my hips broader, and my legs
completely shapeless. Yet the actual traced side
angers me more than my perception, because
it confirms that I am not a shapeless entity.
My waist curves in and my hip curves out.
Tracy claims that a woman is proportional if
her shoulder aligns with her hip. Mine align
perfectly, but I still hate my body.

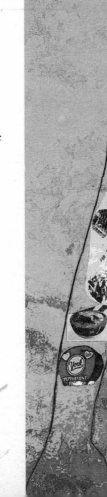

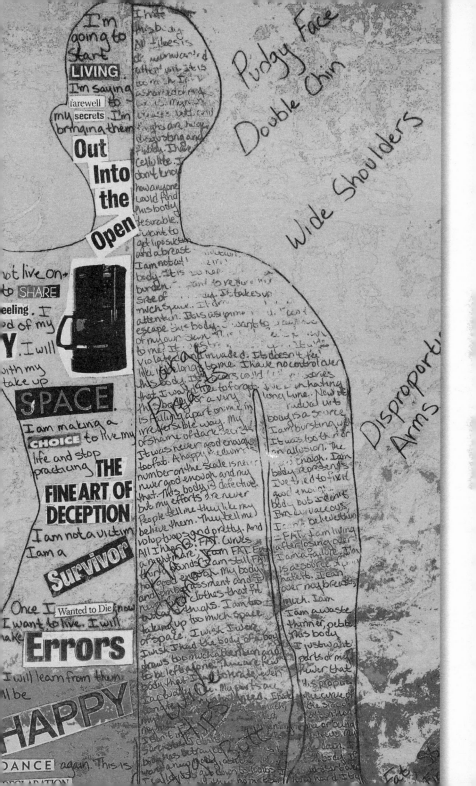

The Full Body Trace project will go much better. I will do it the week I discharge, whereas the Half Perception/Half Trace occurs halfway through my eighty-eight-day stay. Something clicks for me when I look at my body outline on the paper. I realize with a sense of shock that I have been completely ridiculous. The body on the paper is not so bad; it has curves, but proportional ones. It is not the thinnest body, but it is not overly large. For the first time in years, I see through the veil of my eating-disordered perception, if only for a few minutes. And I start to cry when I think about all the time I've wasted trying to reduce and diminish the perfectly good body on the paper before me.

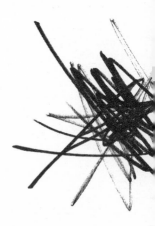

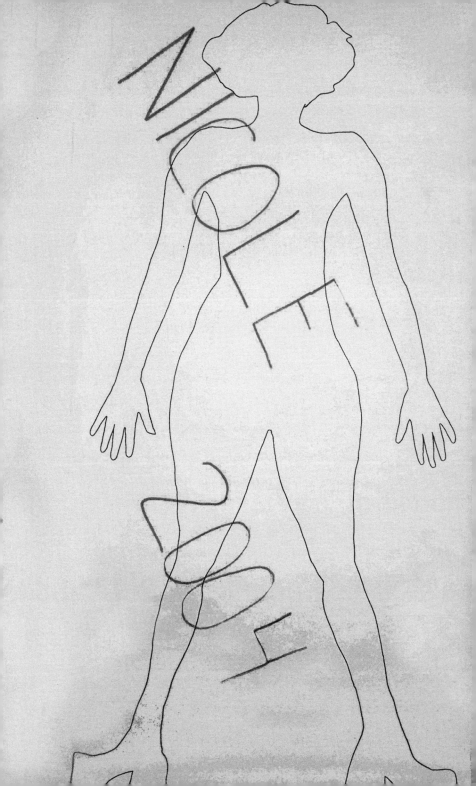

Thin Clothes Bonfire

Tracy tells us to bring our thin clothes to Art Therapy because we are going to burn them. Everyone tells me to bring my favorite size 9 jeans, the ones I have hopes of fitting into again someday. Soon after the day I writhed around on the floor, bemoaning their growing tightness, I had to stop wearing them. But I can't bear to watch them burn, so they sit in the back of my closet, a reminder of my thinner days. The RCs tell me they are my eating disorder jeans, but I don't care. In the end, they will fit me again.

They are Mossimo brand, low-rise, flare-leg jeans. I bought them at SuperTarget on Nicollet Mall in Minneapolis on a golden autumn day, the same day I bought my scale.

The indigo dye has faded with time and washings, and the fabric feels soft and worn-in. The bottoms of the cuffs and the inseam have grown ragged with almost constant wear. At some point the inseam will tear and I will mourn the loss of these perfect jeans.

These jeans are a testament to my personal history. I wore them when I taught class, when I sat in shady bars drinking gin and tonics. Diana, my first girlfriend, often placed her hands in the back pockets of these jeans when we made out.

These jeans have known Minnesota winters, Wisconsin and Pennsylvania summers.

They are the jeans I wore at the height of my eating disorder. At first they were almost too snug, and then they grew so baggy that I couldn't wear them without a belt.

The pockets of these jeans have held dollars, miscellaneous change, phone numbers, lip gloss, condoms, tampons, my cell phone, shopping lists, and ticket stubs.

These jeans, a vestige of my eating disorder, have been through so much with me that I just can't let go.

Laura burns her black polyester thong; it emits a foul, synthetic odor as it smokes and smolders. Danielle burns letters that she wrote to her anorexia. Holly burns a shirt and pair of pants that are now too small. Sarah and Courtney aren't ready to let go yet, so they just sit and watch everything burn.

I take a pastel purple tank top to the Thin Clothes Bonfire. I don't usually wear pastels, but I went through a phase when I was determined to wear lighter colors. But I felt out of place in the pastel tank top, as if it belonged to some sorority sister with a swinging blond ponytail and a butterfly tattoo. As I toss the tank top into the bonfire, Tracy asks what it symbolizes. I say: the girl who was never good enough, the girl everyone else wanted me to be, the girl I will never be. I stare into the fire and watch as my symbolic ideal of myself vanishes into smoke and embers.

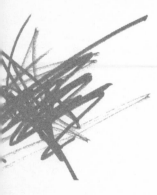

BELONGINGS RUN

There is a designated day for each floor's/unit to go to the designated store to pick up personal belongings needed for the week. Belongings- run is done on a BI-weekly basis (with the exception of the adolescent foor).

The following stores have been approved for belongings run:
Wal-Mart, Target, and K-Mart.
Resident's and staff will decide which store the belongings run will take place.

Belongings run **can not** be done at Kohl's, Goodwill, Bath and Body works etc. etc.

Resident ability to participate in the outing is determined by the treatment team. Residents on ORANGE, RED or OBSERVATION level **may not** participate in the belongings run. Residents must be on YELLOW or GREEN to participate.

The belongings run **is not** to be used as a "shopping spree". This outing is designed to give the residents an opportunity to pick up essential items that they need.

Residents will be given **1-hour only** *(no exceptions)* in the store, and this includes checkout time, so please plan your time wisely. RCs have the option of pulling the next outing if residents are disrespectful or do not follow the guidelines. *Per RC discretion.* RCs can stop the outing at any time if residents are seen with contraband or not following the buddy guidelines. Adolescents must stay with staff at all times.

No other stops will be made other than to the store that is chosen. *(i.e. no stopping at the gas station for cigarettes).*

If residents are unable to participate in this outing, they may give a peer money to purchase any items that they will need for the week. (Note: Adult residents may not purchase cigarettes for adolescent residents at any time. Cigarettes that are applied to minors will be thrown away immediately.)

All residents must have their bags checked upon return from the outing.

Black Market and Contraband

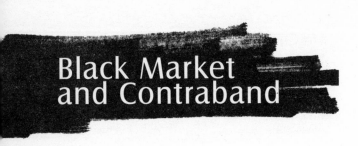

Sharps (razor, tweezers, nail clippers), products containing alcohol (hairspray, perfume), mirrors, and my cell phone—all of these items are kept in my personal bin in the office. They must be signed out by an RC. I have signed away my right to shave my legs whenever I want, as well as to use my cell phone before 4:00 PM.

Upon my arrival, my economy-size bottle of Metabolife diet pills is confiscated. I never see it again.

I discover that there is a thriving black market at the EDC. Gum is the most popular item, as it is small and easy to conceal in a padded bra (just remove the padding) or in the sole of a shoe. Diet Coke is also popular, but rarer, as it is hard to sneak in unless the smuggler is wearing a hooded sweatshirt with a big pocket in the front. It is summer when I am at the EDC, so wearing sweatshirts arouses suspicion. Diet Coke smuggling is on a decline until fall.

Laura is a candy fiend. Her side of the room contains bag upon bag of candy, Lorna Doones, and Diet Coke hidden between her mattress and bed frame. After her off-campus Alcoholics Anonymous meetings three evenings a week, she tosses the contraband up to the deck, where she retrieves it after checking in for the night. I later learn her AA sponsor is buying bagloads of candy for Laura to sneak into the EDC.

One night when Laura is out, I decide to steal a piece of chocolate from her secret stash. Just one piece, because it's there and I don't know when I will have the opportunity to eat chocolate again. I savor the texture of rich, dark chocolate, letting it dissolve into nothingness in my mouth. I take another piece and repeat the process until I have eaten the entire bar. I read the nutritional information on the wrapper and contemplate purging. I decide not to, to see what it feels like to eat something rich and not purge.

Danielle sneaks into my room while Laura is out on pass and I am sitting in the office, talking to RC Caroline. Danielle binges on Butterfingers and Jolly Ranchers, then purges. Later that night, she confesses and I raid Laura's side of the room, gathering up bags of contraband that I give to RC Caroline, who has grown disgusted with Laura.

I have partaken in the gum chewing and diet soda guzzling and binged on candy because the opportunity to have these forbidden things doesn't arise every day. These actions lead to my chugging a liter of Diet Code Red Mountain Dew while I am on pass. I come back to the floor a jittery, wild-eyed mess.

Moderation was never a concept that I practiced. The eating-disordered are infamous for all-or-nothing thinking and impulsivity.

During a trip to the Milwaukee Art Museum, Sandra and I slip into the café and order coffee and Diet Coke that we must drink within a few minutes, before the RCs and Art Therapist Tracy realize we are gone. The van ride back to the EDC is miserable. The air-conditioning is broken and the temperature is in the upper eighties. Traffic has slowed to a rush-hour crawl on I-94. The coffee and Diet Coke are roiling in my stomach, which has forgotten how to deal with large quantities of caffeine. I spend my evening retching over the toilet, so miserable that I use my skills at purging to make myself vomit and feel better (plus, it's an excuse to purge).

Weekly trips to Target and the local movie theater present a tempting opportunity to consume contraband. At Target, a resident "takes one for the team" and distracts the RC who is with us on the belongings run (our biweekly trip to buy necessities at Target or Wal-Mart that often turns into a giddy, contraband-filled shopping spree). Then someone else buys diet soda in the express aisle and carries it around the store in her purse. We chug soda in the automotive section, hidden among car batteries and windshield fluid. We eat candy in the lingerie section, ducking beneath boy-cut briefs.

At the movie theater, we are permitted one small popcorn as a snack challenge and one small soda that is neither caffeinated nor diet. After the lights dim, we exchange our Sprite for Diet Coke and buy Sno-Caps and Reese's Pieces. We munch away happily and slurp our soda slowly during the movie, making it last as long as possible.

Knowing My Weight

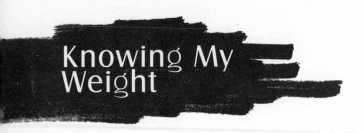

"Give me one good reason to tell you your weight," says Dietitian Caroline.

She stares at me with skeptical eyes. I curl my body into a ball on the sofa, enveloped in the afghan my great-aunt crocheted for my high school graduation. At the EDC it has become my security blanket and a way of hiding my body.

"If you tell me my weight, I won't believe that I weigh three hundred pounds. It will be a reality check."

I've become very good at manipulating staff during my time at the EDC.

Dietitian Caroline sighs as she opens the pink binder to my weight-and-vitals page. We have this conversation every time we meet.

"You're at 139 pounds. That's stable and within your weight range."

"I've gained eight pounds since I've been here; how is that stable?" I ask.

"You're going through the refeeding process; everyone gains some weight," says Dietitian Caroline.

I smile sweetly at Dietitian Caroline and leave the conference room, careful not to slam the glass door behind me. I fling myself onto my bed and cocoon the covers around me, even though it's about eighty degrees in my room. I begin kicking my legs and wailing with histrionic sobs. I resolve never to leave my narrow hospital bed—139 is almost 140, and 140 is almost 150, which is three-quarters of the way to 200. And that is fat.

Laura bursts into our room, ruddy-cheeked from a climb on the ropes course. She hears my muffled snuffling.

"Nicole, why are you crying? It's too hot to hide under the covers."

Laura crawls into bed with me and I gasp, "139," and Laura snuggles against me and murmurs comforting words in my ear. I begin raving, declaring that Dietitian Caroline is a sadist, that the Wisconsin Department of Health needs to shut this place down, and that I'm going on a hunger strike because I hate my body and hate my life.

Laura untangles herself from my sweaty covers and returns with Alistair, her stuffed dog. She places him in the crook of my arm.

Dietitian Caroline comes into the room and hovers over my bed.

"I knew this was going to happen. This is not an excuse for you to purge," she says.

Later that day, after a dinner of four-cheese lasagna, I slip down the hall and into the bathroom and hork up my dinner. I almost choke on rubbery globs of semidigested lasagna, and the whole time I'm purging I am filled with hatred I will never be rid of.

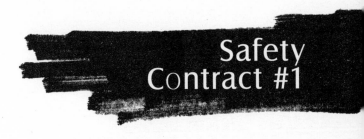

Safety
Contract #1

I, NICOLE JOHNS, *promise not to purge*
for the remainder of the night. If I am
having urges, I will find an RC and
talk about why I want to purge.
I will stay safe tonight.

i will stay safe tonight.

Periods

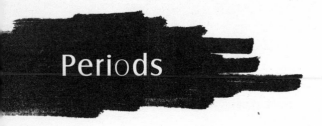

out half of us still menstruate

About half of us still menstruate. Most of us who do are
bulimics or EDNOS. We are generally not emaciated like our
anorexic counterparts, who lack enough body fat to menstruate.
In fact, we are more likely to be overweight than underweight.

The anorexics view their menstrual cycles as a dreaded curse. If
they weigh enough to menstruate, they believe they are fat.

I never lose my period. It is light and irregular for a while, but
it never disappears.

Then it starts getting heavier as I gain weight and grow
healthier. It is all I can talk about when I have it, maybe because
it is a sign of health. We are period-obsessed, talking about the

duration of our cycles, whether we have cramps, and what our favorite method of feminine protection is.

In Psychodrama, we have to pick a sheer colored fabric that represents how we feel. I pick bright red and wrap it around me like a crimson cocoon.

Fat Is Not a Feeling

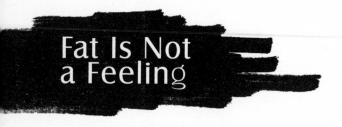

art therapy (and most other

In Art Therapy (and most other forms of Group Therapy),
we rate our body image on a scale of one to ten, with ten being
fantastic and one being horrible. In addition to assigning our body
image a numerical value, we pick an adjective to describe how we
are feeling. To help us with this task, Art Therapist Tracy has
created a colorful construction paper–and-marker list of adjectives
for us to choose from. We take turns going around the table and
checking in with Tracy about how we are feeling. A typical check-
in goes like this:

LAURA: I'm feeling like a fucking negative twenty today and I feel angry and hurt.

HOLLY: Oh, I'm about a four with body image and I feel content.

SANDRA: My body image is a six and I feel . . . a lot of feelings.

ELIZA: I'm about a seven today and I feel creative.

ME: My body image is a two and I feel fat.

"Fat is not a feeling, Nicole," says Tracy.

"But I feel fat."

"You need to explore what is making you feel dissatisfied with your body image," says Tracy.

How do you explain to someone—who has never had an eating disorder—that fat is a feeling?

To be more precise, fat is a combination of feelings and experiences. It is a complex feeling, a collection of simple feelings bound together. I notice my body more when I am in an uncomfortable situation, when I am emotionally overstimulated or fearful. By focusing on my body at the precise moment when I am so emotionally uncomfortable, I am deflecting the uncomfortable emotions onto something more tangible—my body. When I say I'm feeling fat, I am eluding my feelings; it is a defense mechanism.

"Fat" has become my standard response when someone in the therapeutic world asks me how I'm feeling. Most of the time I can't even (or don't want to) figure out what I am feeling. So instead

I focus on the circumference of my thigh, the heaviness of my breasts, the double chin I swear I saw in the mirror this morning. Like all addicts, the eating-disordered person goes to great lengths to avoid her feelings.

"Fat" is code for feeling scared, angry, ashamed, hurt, and sad all in one. It is code for I don't want to talk about it; just leave me alone.

Dairy Queen

We are standing in line at Dairy Queen, pondering what to
order. There are six of us on this outing, eight if you include RC
Julia and RC Marie. We know the rules: Whatever we get must
have ice cream in it, and it can't be larger than a medium. Some
of us eye the illuminated menu with lusty, ravenous eyes; we want
everything, even though it won't satiate us. The rest of us dread the
taste of vanilla; we are thinking that ice cream is made with cream
and cream is not something we allow ourselves to eat.

I fall between the two extremes. I am afraid that if I eat one ice
cream cone, I will want another and another and then will have to
make myself sick to get rid of all the calories. This outing is

supposed to show us that we can eat ice cream in moderation, and that it won't make us gain weight instantaneously. Everyone else is ordering small Blizzards, so I order a small Toffee Cheesecake Blizzard, even though I don't really like Blizzards.

We sit on a long green bench outside Dairy Queen while nibbling our cones and nervously scooping spoonfuls of Blizzard into our mouths. RC Julia and RC Marie sit inside at a booth where they can see us. To distract ourselves, we play a game Eliza has taught us: Friend, Fuck, Push Off a Cliff. The premise is that one person picks three celebrities and another person has to decide whom they'd pick as their friend, whom they would fuck, and whom they would push off a cliff. Everyone wants to push Michael Jackson off a cliff and fuck Brad Pitt.

I eat one-third of my Blizzard and impulsively toss it into the garbage can because I know if I eat the rest of it, I will have to purge later. Some of the other women eat their Blizzards, some don't.

On the way back to the EDC, we sit in Big Red and play the Friend, Fuck, Push Off a Cliff game some more. We even get RC Julia and RC Marie to play, and we laugh and try not to think about the ice cream sitting in our stomachs, about the calories and fat grams floating in our malnourished bodies. Instead, we laugh and watch the sun set over the cornfields of southeast Wisconsin.

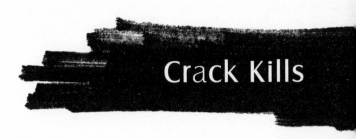

Crack Kills

evan is a muscular
x-foot-two firefighter

RC Evan is a muscular, six-foot-two firefighter who also works at the EDC. Evan and I bond over the fact that we are both originally from western Pennsylvania. Like me, he finds Midwesterners a bit ridiculous, with their strange accents and closed-off personalities. We talk about the Steelers and the Pirates. We talk about how Pittsburgh has cleaned up a lot.

One of RC Evan's favorite pastimes is picking on Holly. A typical conversation between them goes like this:

Holly: I need my meds.

Evan (smirking): Can you ask politely?

Holly: I need my fucking meds. Now.

Evan: Inappropriate, Holly, simply inappropriate.

Holly: Fucking shit, what is your problem? You're inappropriate, Mr. Firefighter.

Eventually RC Evan will give Holly her meds and Holly will pretend to be pissed, but she'll sit down in the office with RC Evan and me, where we always ask him if he's fought any fires recently, if his incredibly jealous and nosy girlfriend (whom we've dubbed the CIA) is still riding his ass, and how his kids are doing.

At some point during our conversation, RC Evan will open a drawer in the filing cabinet and pull out a package of jawbreakers. He'll pop one into his mouth and crack a big, gap-toothed smile while Holly and I complain about how inappropriate it is for a staff member to be eating candy in front of a resident. RC Evan will just lean back in his chair and smile the whole time.

Holly and I know we are RC Evan's favorite residents long before he ever confirms it. We are spirited and wild, unlike the anorexics, but we aren't as crazy as Laura or Sandra.

One anonymous night in early July, when Natalie comes in for the night shift, she bends over to pick something up, with her backside facing RC Evan and Holly.

"Did you know that crack kills, Natalie?" says Holly.

RC Evan almost swallows his jawbreaker.

"Holly, you are just so strange," says Natalie.

RC Evan and I leave the office and go out to the deck, where we erupt in laughter. Holly joins us and coolly smokes a cigarette.

Later, when I am close to discharge, RC Evan will start slipping me candy when no one is watching. I will like that we are breaking the rules, and that he thinks I can handle having candy without purging.

Holly starts a fire in one of the industrial-size ashtrays on the deck to keep her hands warm while she smokes. RC Evan smells the smoke and sprints to the deck, ready to fight a fire. Instead, he finds Holly puffing away happily in front of her own private flame.

"No fires! We don't have fires at the EDC!" Evan yells, as Holly laughs.

After that, whenever Evan works, Holly runs around the day-room shouting that there are no fires at the EDC, while Evan shakes his head at her inappropriateness.

After I discharge from the EDC, I fly home to Pennsylvania and drive back to Minnesota. Holly flies out to Pennsylvania to road-trip with me because she has never been out east. We decide to take a detour in Wisconsin. We call Evan at the EDC, and he tells us to meet him there after his shift. For a couple hours, we catch up and joke with him.

Before we leave, he tells us that he is proud of us.

RC Evan tells us we are going to make it.

And we believe him.

Voodoo House Field Trip

we become obsessed with We've become obsessed with the Voodoo House on County Road P. RC Julia showed it to us on our way back from a trip to Target. She slowed the van to a crawl as we plastered our faces against the windows, trying to get a better look at the ruby-red stained glass windows, stick figures hanging from the porch, and creepy devil sculptures in the front yard. We begged Julia to pull over and let us out to look at it, but she kept driving.

The next time we go out, we convince Julia to park the van at a wayside so we can walk up to the Voodoo House for a better look. Seven of us walk single file up the road, with Laura leading the line and RC Julia at the end. We stare at the devil statues, stick figures, and cryptic symbols that adorn the Voodoo House. We disregard the no trespassing signs that are posted liberally around the yard. Someone in the Voodoo House is watching *Friends*; we can see the flickering of the television and hear Jennifer Aniston arguing with Courteney Cox.

Laura, our daredevil ringleader, is exploring the front yard. Julia hisses at her to come back. We hear voices and take off down the road, abandoning Laura. Back at the van, we see that RC Julia has gotten a ticket for parking illegally in what was really a boat launch, not a wayside.

Fight Club

starts with the manic need

It starts with the manic need to rearrange the dayroom furniture. After we shove the worn sofas into the corners, vacuum the rug, and dust the end tables and mantel (and burn some calories), we survey the rearranged, clean dayroom. Earlier in the day, we decided to institute EDC Fight Club to liven up the evening. The first match would be me versus Holly.

During Art Therapy we make posters advertising the impending Fight Club. Holly's Fight Club alias is Smokey McSmokerson because of the large quantities of cigarettes she smokes, and I am dubbed Bookish Babe because of my propensity to curl up on the sofa with a book during any free time. Fight Club is scheduled to begin at 7:00 PM, and the admission cost is one cigarette, which is to be given to Smokey McSmokerson.

RC Julia and RC Camille are working tonight. They sit in the office, chatting with each other. By staying in the office while we manically rearrange the dayroom and institute Fight Club, they are condoning our behavior. Later, Julia tells me Fight Club is a good idea because it releases some of our frenzied negative energy.

Holly and I clear the center floor space while the other residents choose seats and ready their cameras. Laura is officiating; she tells us she wants to see a good clean fight, and then it's on.

We circle each other and make karate-chop motions. Courtney sneaks over to the stereo and starts blaring "Bombs over Baghdad," by OutKast, while everyone else is laying bets on who will win. Most people bet on Holly, since she is a good four inches taller than I am. But when she starts posing for the cameras, I seize the opportunity to jump on her and take her down. We both tumble to the floor and I crawl on top of Holly, pinning her arms with my knees, while she bellows that I don't fight fair (she claims I smothered her with my breasts; I did not), even as she bites my forearm. Laura proclaims me the winner and says she wants to fight me next, and Eliza says she'll challenge Holly. RC Julia watches the whole thing from the doorway of the office and is smiling and shaking her head.

"I had no idea you were so vicious, Miss Nicole. I didn't think you had it in you," she says.

Laura is harder to take down. She is wiry and strong; she keeps slipping out of my grasp. But eventually, I take her down too. Holly wins the fight against Eliza because Eliza can't stop laughing. Fight Club is deemed successful, but the next morning Therapist Elaine outlaws any further rumbles, on the basis that we are exercising and someone is bound to get hurt.

When I show RC Julia the bite mark Holly has left on my forearm, her eyes grow large and she tells me that Wisconsin law requires that I get an AIDS test, since Holly and I have exchanged fluids. I tell her everything is fine because Holly hasn't broken my skin. I wear my Penn State sweatshirt until the bite marks fade.

Danielle and I try instituting EDC Dance Party the next night, grinding against each other while bad '90s techno music reverberates through the dayroom, but RC Camille thinks we are exercising.

EDC Arm Wrestling entertains us for one dull afternoon. Staff even gets in on the action. Dietitian Caroline is beaten easily, while RC Allison beats us all and proclaims herself champion. Therapist Elaine just shakes her head from the sidelines.

Team Building

Laura kicks the wall five times during a manic episode (she has bipolar disorder) because Sandra claims that Laura's smoking near the patio door has irritated her asthma. Instead of kicking Sandra, Laura kicks the wall, bruising her toes badly, and spends the afternoon in the local ER, happily sipping diet soda while having her foot wrapped and enjoying a Darvocet-induced haze. The result is an additional Group Therapy session during which everyone is anti-Sandra and staff cracks down on the cliques that have formed within the group.

Clique number one (the aggressive, dominant, bulimic clique): Holly, Laura, me. We tear around the EDC, yelling about how miserable we are and blowing everything up into a major drama. When Holly loses her cigarettes, she plops down in front of the office and rolls around on the floor, laughing and screaming, "I can't find my cigarettes! Somebody stole my cigarettes! I'm going to die!" One night in the middle of July, Laura duct tapes all my belongings, including the sheets on my bed. I laugh and duct tape her shirt, as well as Holly's. Laura also puts Holly's teddy bear in a noose she creates from duct tape, and hangs the bear prominently in the dayroom; this prank upsets Eliza, who had a friend who committed suicide via hanging.

While technically part of the bulimic clique, I am often too caught up in my own misery to effectively incite mayhem on our floor. I am too busy tossing my snack off the deck when no one is looking, sneaking down the hall to purge during some drama on the floor after dinner, or changing my clothes thirteen times a day because I believe they all make me look fat.

During a gynecology consult, I step on the scale when the nurse isn't watching and move the bars around until they are even and I know my weight. At the same consult, as soon as the nurse leaves the room for me to change, I hide my snack of oyster crackers deep in the trash can filled with medical waste.

Once I learn that team-building activities are imminent, I voice my opinion rather loudly.

"Team building makes me hate myself," I yell.

"You really need to work on your attitude today," says RC Shannon. I give her the finger once she turns around.

Clique number two (the passive, submissive, mostly anorexic clique): Eliza, Danielle, Sandra. They go to bed at 9:00 PM and mostly sit on the sofas and knit. The bulimic clique's boisterousness makes them nervous.

We are supposed to go to a Milwaukee Brewers game tonight, but Therapist Elaine thinks it's a good idea to do team-building activities instead, to facilitate a better group dynamic and erode some of the bulimic clique's power.

I have been looking forward to the Brewers game for weeks. Baseball reminds me of summer evenings as a child, driving to Three Rivers Stadium in Pittsburgh to watch the Pirates play, back when they were good. Baseball games were happy times when I ate popcorn, watched fireworks, and tailgated with my family.

Team-building activities are scheduled for after dinner. I simmer with anger all through dinner; I can barely swallow my Cuban black bean casserole. After dinner we sit on the porch and smoke, while talking about boycotting team building. The program motto is "Challenge by choice," and we are ready to choose.

"What the fuck are they going to make us do, sing 'Kumbaya' and hold hands?" asks Holly.

We make up our own version of "Kumbaya." It goes like this: "Kumbaya, this blows, suck my ass. Kumbaya, this blows, suck my ass. Oh, Shannon, suck my ass."

Therapist Elaine overhears us and is not pleased. We get a lecture about positive attitude.

After slamming the patio door so hard the glass shakes, Holly and I go into the dayroom. RC Shannon and RC Julia take us out to the parking lot and have us all line up single file, with our hands on the person's shoulders in front of us. We have to come up with a team name, and someone picks Camp Turtle Pond for the Nutritionally Challenged, which is shortened to Team Turtle. We all have to hop in sync and shout, "Team Turtle," and if someone is out of sync or refuses to participate, we have to go back to the beginning.

I refuse to say "Team Turtle." We go back to the beginning.

Here I am, twenty-three years old and forced to participate in some ridiculous team-building activity. I am absolutely livid with pent-up rage. I manage to mutter "Team Turtle" and hop, just so we can get the activity over with.

Back inside, Shannon and Julia make us all hold hands and twist into a messed-up circle. We are supposed to work together to untangle ourselves. The whole scene feels unreal; I am so angry that I am calm. After we untangle ourselves, we are sent to our rooms to pick a song that symbolizes a happy time for us. I know this is dangerous territory.

I pick the song "Wildflowers" by Tom Petty because it reminds me of the spring days at the end of my senior year of college that I spent driving around Lake Erie with my ex-boyfriend Jordan. It was a time when I was not actively eating-disordered; I stopped purging when I started dating Jordan. I was happy with my life then. Jordan used to sing "Wildflowers" to me, emphasizing the lyric "You belong with your love on your arm, you belong somewhere you feel free."

I left Jordan when I left Pennsylvania.

We play our favorite songs for the whole group. Some residents have Christian songs, others hard rock. I am fine until Danielle puts on "My Immortal" by Evanescence. I start wailing. I curl into a ball on the sofa and choke and gasp and heave. Laura tries to wipe my nose, Holly puts her arms around me, Eliza smoothes my hair, and Shannon and Julia coax me to play my song. Eliza puts "Wildflowers" on the stereo and I cry harder; it is the kind of crying that hurts your lungs and makes you hysterical with grief that is so built up, you can't even begin to figure out what it's about, much less talk about it.

"Do you want to talk about why you're crying?" asks Julia.

"No."

When I calm down, I apologize for singing the inappropriate version of "Kumbaya," for slamming the patio door so hard the floor shook, and for telling Julia I was "fanfuckintabulous." Shannon and Julia accept my apology and say they are happy I have broken open.

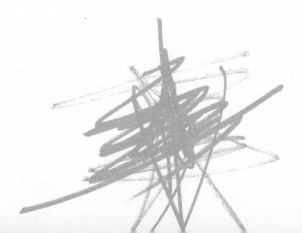

183

184   Purge

SPONTANEOUS
"RC OUTINGS"

Spontaneous *"RC Outings"* were designed by this facility to allow residents t[hat] do not have passes on the weekends (i.e. being from out-of-state and having transportation, or being an adolescent with no access to a vehicle et[c.]) to get some community interaction.

Spontaneous *"RC outings"* are to be decided by the RCs working second shift o[n] Saturday. This is to help the resident *"Let go of some of the contro[l]"*. **Spontaneous outings will not occur every weekend, and may no[t] occur on Friday or Sunday.** *"RC Outings"* will occur under the RC discretion **only**. (i.e. RCs have to look at acuity, staffing, weather, vehicle availability etc). There are many factors that go into the decision making for an *"RC outing"* which can only be made by the RC working that night. Which is why a decision will be made on second shift as to whether there will be a spontaneous *"RC Outing"* that night and not before. If the residents on the floor are doing well, the RC will try to have a *"RC outing"* on Saturday. If a large percentage of the group has passes that weekend – there will probably not be a "RC Outing" on Saturday. **If residents tell the RCs where the outing is going to occur and where the outing is going to be – it will be canceled for that weekend** (i.e. ~~"your taking us to the movies tonight"~~ etc.). Residents need to *"let go"* and trust in the staff's decision. Think of it as *"Blind Outings"*. The RCs may also decide that not going on an outing would be therapeutic for the group? Again it is up to the RCs.

RCs may only choose from **one** of the following destinations: Movie (Hillside, Capitol, Ben Franklin, Library (Waukesha or Oconomowoc), and Barnes & Noble (Brookfield), and the Half Price Bookstore. *(Blockbuster can be added to any of the outings above if there is time).* Permission may be received to go to other places not on the list per RC, treatment team and Administrative discretion.

Spontaneous *"RC outings"* will only be done if there is no programming *(i.e. Rap speaker etc.)* and the staff to resident ratio cannot be greater than 5-1. If the RCs choose to have a *"RC outing"* on Saturday evening and there are some residents that had passes earlier in the day or have a pass on Sunday – they can still participate in the *"RC outing"*.

Playground Love

One boring Saturday night in mid-July, RC Julia and RC Evan ask

us if we want to go on an outing. We say yes, of course. Somehow it

is decided that we will go to a playground, since it is a nice night and

we have a lot of pent-up energy, according to the RCs.

Recreational Therapist Douglas has taken us to this play-

ground before, so that we could let our inner children run wild.

At the playground, Laura heads for the swings, Holly runs for

the fort and proclaims herself queen of the world, and Eliza and I

make our way to the monkey bars with Sandra.

We watch as Sandra, who is wearing a jean skirt, hangs

upside down by her knees, her white granny panties and stick legs fully exposed.

"Hey, Sandra, I can see your underwear," says Eliza.

"Yeah, I know," says Sandra.

"Well, I just thought you should know," says Eliza.

RC Julia comes over to the monkey bars.

"Sandra, I can see your underwear," says RC Julia.

"Yeah, I know," says Sandra.

"Well, that's inappropriate," says RC Julia.

"But I'm just trying to get comfortable with my body," says Sandra.

"You need to get comfortable with it somewhere in private," says RC Julia.

Sandra flips off the monkey bars, and we watch as RC Julia and RC Evan start swinging on the swing set, side by side. We have no basis for our belief that Julia and Evan are having a steamy, sensual affair, but it keeps us amused, so we go with it. We speculate on what they are talking about while they swing.

Once dusk settles over the playground, the RCs round us up and we head back to the EDC. We are wild and raucous; we try to institute Fight Club in the van, and we throw things at RC Evan (we would throw things at RC Julia, but she's driving). We beg RC Julia to drive past the Voodoo House, and she agrees just to shut us up.

Strange, strobelike light beams are emanating from the Voodoo House. Laura jumps out of the van and starts taking pictures, RC Julia yells at Laura and tells RC Evan to go after her, and RC

Evan says no way because the black man is always the first to get killed in these situations. We are all laughing hysterically.

Laura jumps back into the van, breathless and sweaty; we return to the EDC in time for evening snack time; and our carefree mood dissipates quickly.

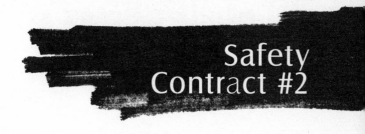

Safety
Contract #2

I, NICOLE JOHNS, *promise not to drink*
more than one cup of coffee and
one caffeinated soda while on pass.
I will not abuse caffeine in an
attempt to dull hunger.

i. nicole johns. promise

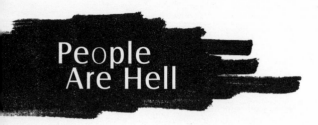

People Are Hell

ople are hell, nicole

"People are hell, Nicole."

That is what Dirk told me as he drove me home after I'd been stranded at his house the night before. Another one of the endless Great Lakes blizzards had put down two feet of lake-effect snow in a matter of hours, and the interstates had been closed.

"Do you know who I'm quoting, Nicole?"

"No," I said as I watched the snow-covered vineyards of northern Pennsylvania fade into the white brightness of the horizon. My breath fogged the window of his Honda Civic.

"Sartre. You really should read some of his work."

I recount this dialogue during Psychodrama with Rachel. I

had told her I wanted to do a psychodrama about the night I spent at Dirk's house, because maybe then I could move on fully from the experience. Despite all the geography between us, the formal request from Penn State Erie that he keep his distance from me, and the years gone by, I can't forget.

Dirk was my senior thesis adviser at Penn State Erie.

He asked me to dog-sit for him.

I said yes.

He invited me to his house after school, so I could see where everything was and meet the dog.

It started snowing.

I had never driven in snow.

Dirk said he would drive.

I said yes.

I met the dog, saw the house.

Dirk started drinking and offered me a glass of wine.

I said no.

He tried to drive me back to Erie. The roads were closed.

He asked me if I wanted a glass of wine.

I said yes.

He told me to pick a bottle from his collection; I picked a French red.

I drank.

We listened to Beth Orton.

I drank.

He topped off my glass.

I drank.

He made me a dinner of pasta with clam sauce.

I ate and I drank.

I told him about the bulimia.

He told me about his recent divorce.

We both drank.

He said he was lonely. He needed friends. He was alone.

I sat on the sofa with him.

We drank.

He said he wanted to be friends.

I started crying.

I blacked out.

I woke up to his hands on my feet, then my calves, then my thighs.

I blacked out.

I woke up propped against his shoulder, my feet on top of his.

He gave me a shirt to sleep in. It was size XXL. Eddie Bauer. Forest green.

My white shirt was stained with red wine.

The next morning, he tells me to keep everything quiet.

He could lose his job.

I tell my friends.

I am infuriated.

I tell members of the English department.

They say to keep quiet.

He doesn't have tenure.

He could lose his job.

I report him to the sexual harassment counselor.

I report him to the head of humanities and social sciences.

He is everywhere.

He asks my friends about me.

He tries to talk to me.

A letter goes in his file.

A restraining order is issued.

I am told to keep quiet.

I am told how mature I am for not seeking revenge.

I graduate and move to Minnesota.

I don't have to keep quiet anymore.

The years of silence choke me. The first event I write about when I move to Minnesota is the Dirk ordeal because, finally, I can speak freely. From the night I spent at his house until the day I graduated from Penn State Erie, my eating disorder worsened. I was symbolically stuffing my feelings and then purging them, since speaking about them was forbidden. Even after I move to Minnesota, the blank spaces in my mind bother me. What happened during the times I blacked out? Was I manhandled or raped? I believe I would've known if I had been violated, but doubt creeps into my mind. I was still dressed, I reassure myself. But I will never know the truth.

I tell Rachel all of this. I tell her I want to do a psychodrama about Dirk, because maybe that way I will be able to move on. She agrees that it's a good idea.

Rachel asks me to arrange the room like I usually have my classroom arranged when I teach Introduction to Creative Writing at the University of Minnesota. I arrange all the chairs in a circle, and all the residents, my simulated students, pick a seat. Rachel tells the students to ask me about what books I've read. Laura asks me if I've ever read Tolstoy's *War and Peace*.

I say no.

"What kind of teacher are you if you've never even read *War and Peace?*" asks Rachel.

"A perfectly fine one. No one has read all the classics," I reply.

"Everyone, I want you to pretend you are Nicole's students. Give her a hard time about her not having read *War and Peace*, and just harass her in general," says Rachel.

"You suck as a teacher."

"You're only twenty-three; how can you teach college?"

"I'm better read than you."

"Just who the hell do you think you are?"

I listen to these voices and decide this whole tableau would never occur in real life. The classroom is one of the places where I feel most comfortable. It is a place where I can forget that I have an eating disorder. And I always get wonderful student evaluations. But I decide to play along with Rachel.

"You're not good enough."

"You aren't thin."

Now my students are interjecting issues from a recent Group Therapy session, also something that would never happen in real life.

"Rachel, this would never happen in real life. I'm completely comfortable in the classroom," I say.

Rachel calls an end to the scene and has me arrange the furniture in the same way Dirk's living room was arranged. I am not feeling anything other than anger at what I deem Rachel's ineptitude. There is no sense of catharsis in this psychodrama. Instead, I feel my cheeks begin to burn with anger. This is not helping. Nothing will ever help. True, I am holding back—I'm not surrendering to treatment. But I've surrendered before, and it has only gotten me into bad situations.

We act out the evening at Dirk's, with Holly playing Dirk.

Rachel has Dirk stand behind me and cover my eyes. I just stand there, not sure what to do.

"Why don't you fight back, Nicole?" asks Rachel.

"I don't know," I reply. I know where this is heading, and I don't like it.

You are not blowing aimlessly in the wind. You have control.

I fight Holly off.

"Why were you drinking?" asks Rachel.

"I don't know."

"You blacked out, correct?"

"Yes."

"Alcoholics black out."

Silence.

"I am not an alcoholic."

I am fiery with silent rage. Alcoholics are physically addicted to alcohol. I am not.

"Would this have happened had you not been drinking?" asks Rachel.

I am itching to punch Rachel smack in her pointy face.

"You are resisting the psychodrama; you are not letting go."

I have no response to this comment. Psychodrama ends, and we file upstairs for dinner. RC Julia attended my psychodrama; I asked her to come, since I thought I'd have a hard time. At dinner, she sits at my table.

"How do you think that went?" she asks as she butters her roll.

"Terribly. I'm not an alcoholic, and I don't appreciate Rachel intimating that everything was my fault."

RC Julia doesn't know what to say.

"That's some major bullshit," says Holly.

"What if your drink was roofied?" asks Eliza.

"I fucking hate Rachel. She has no idea what she's doing," says Laura.

RC Julia still doesn't know what to say. She just looks at me with what I assume are sympathetic eyes.

"You should confront her," says RC Julia.

"I don't want to. I just want to forget about it," I say.

After dinner, I talk to RC Marie in the office. I tell her about my psychodrama, and she says she has an assignment for me. Intrigued, I ask her what it is. I secretly like assignments because they make me feel like I'm in school.

"I want you to write a letter to Dirk."

I like this idea.

I head down to the conference room with my CD player and listen to Tori Amos's *Little Earthquakes* album, and write a furious letter stained with my angry tears. I feel relief. I feel catharsis. I thank RC Marie and vow to read the letter out loud in Group Therapy the next day.

Laura talks about how she has no choices in her life, and I fidget and sigh during Group Therapy. Finally, I interject.

"Elaine, I really, really need to read this letter."

Laura pouts and becomes silent, and I begin to read.

> *Dirk,*
>
> *I fucking hate you. I hate how you tried to blow the whole incident off, how you pretended to act contrite and said all the right things. I hate how you made my senior year at Penn State Erie such a trial.*
>
> *Do you know what it's like to have anxiety attacks and be so scared that you hide in the bathroom? Because that is what I did. And you kept trying to talk to me. You kept trying to keep me quiet and now I feel like I'm going to fucking explode because I'm so sick of everyone trying to keep me quiet.*
>
> *When you touched me, I wanted to crawl out of my skin. I wanted to die. The thought of your hands on my thighs makes me sick. You worked a bad situation to your advantage and I've been blaming myself.*
>
> *I was not the one who kept filling my wine glass, I did not ask you or want you to touch me. I did not want you. You violated me.*
>
> *I'm so angry that as I write this I can barely contain myself. And maybe I don't want to anymore.*
>
> *Some people have suggested that you put Rohypnol in my drink because I blacked out so suddenly. I don't even want to think about that. I drive myself crazy*

wondering what happened in the blank spaces even though the parts I remember are bad enough.

You not only affected me emotionally, but also academically. You were already my second thesis adviser and because you couldn't keep your lecherous hands to yourself I had three thesis advisers before I finished the damn thing.

I fucking despise how you played innocent when I informed you that you were no longer my adviser.

I fucking hate how you tried to manipulate me, how you tried to appease me, tried to placate me.

I fucking hate how you stared at me while I read from my senior thesis at the English Department Banquet.

And the day you pulled out behind me in the parking lot, I thought you were following me. I want you to know that kind of fear.

In fact, I want you to be stuck in the situation I was in and wake up with some man's hands on your vulnerable thighs. I want you to have to live with the blank spaces in your memory, to keep trying to piece it all together, to play the whole night on repeat in your head.

Most of all I want the memory of a man's hands caressing their way up your thighs to be imprinted in your body and mind. I want you to feel dirty and ashamed. I want you to have to inspect your body for bruises and signs of assault the next day.

Most of all I want you to question what happened in those blank spaces, because that is what torments me.

Wait, I take that back. I fucking want you to become a raging bulimic. I want you to spend days consuming and purging. I want you to isolate yourself from others. I want you to live on a diet of coffee, Diet Coke, and diet pills. I want you to pass out, get concussions, develop heart problems, and pray for death because you are so fucking miserable.

I want you to move halfway across the country and still not be able to forget.

I want you to be ashamed of your body, to hide in sweatshirts and pajama pants.

I want you to hate yourself.

Oh, and another thing, I want you to have to go through the ordeal of filing a sexual harassment complaint. I want everyone to try and keep you quiet. I want you to have to tell your story a minimum of five times. I want you to turn fuchsia each time you tell it.

I want the sexual harassment counselor to tell you how fucking mature you are because you are cooperating and keeping a secret when in reality you want to tell the whole school. I want you to be pressured into signing all the forms.

I hope I never have to see you again. If I do, I will stare you down. You have no power over me now.

So this is all I have to say for now. I'm done being scared and now I'm fucking pissed. You're lucky we're not in the same state because if I was, I'd slash the tires on your lame-ass Honda Civic.

I'm done keeping secrets. I'm tired of taking one for the team and being the peacemaker. That's not me. It never was. The cost of keeping quiet was too high.

I'm done with you.

—NICOLE

As soon as I finish the last sentence, everyone shouts and exclaims that my letter is awesome. RC Allison is especially proud. She jumps out of her seat with a big smile on her face, and I think I detect tears in her eyes. Everyone hugs me. My anger has dissipated, at least for now.

Later that day I talk to Rachel about how angry Psychodrama made me.

"You made me feel like an alcoholic, and like what happened that night was my fault," I say.

"I want you to see that you aren't helpless, that you have control over your life. I don't want you to wallow in victimhood."

"I understand that, but you went about it the wrong way."

"You could have told me to stop; you have the power to do that."

"I didn't think it worked like that," I say.

"The power is always yours," says Rachel.

I try not to hold a grudge against Rachel, but I have lost trust in her. I am skeptical of her methods, and of Psychodrama in general.

Evoking Emotion

IN THE UNEMOTIONAL

Rachel thinks I have been avoiding the ropes course, that I
am harboring a secret fear of heights (in reality, it has been a rainy
summer, and Recreational Therapy has been indoors). She thinks
that if she gets me up in the air, balancing across an inclined log
with nothing to hold on to, my inner emotions will be evoked in this
precarious state. Rachel wants me to feel vulnerable. I want to tell
her to bring it on, that it will take much more than a jaunt up an
inclined log thirty feet in the air to break me.

Thursday comes around, and it's time for this special session of
Psychodrama on the ropes course, otherwise known as Get Nicole
in Touch with Her Feelings Time. It's a balmy August day, and

not many of the residents come to this special Psychodrama (Psy-chotrauma), as they prefer to doze in the murky, arctic chill of the over-air-conditioned and dimly lit dayroom.

Laura is here, though, as are Sarah, Danielle, Sandra, and some girls from the adolescent floor. When I begin my climb up the ladder to the inclined log, Rachel has the other residents shout negative things to me, such as "You aren't good enough, you're never going to make it, you're gaining weight, you have no control." This is supposed to represent my negative voice, the voice of EDNOS that often haunts my head. I tune the voices out and scamper nimbly up the ladder. I spent my childhood climbing trees, so the ladder climb is effortless.

I reach the lower part of the inclined log and stand there for a second, as directed by Rachel.

"How do you feel, Nicole?" she asks.

"Strong, powerful," I say.

"Are you scared that you are up so high?"

"No, it's great; the view up here is amazing."

"Continue on, then."

I extend my arms out to the side for balance. I pretend I am ten years old again, walking across the balance beam at gymnastics practice, putting one foot in front of the other and holding my arms out gracefully. I make it easily to the middle of the log, where Rachel has me stop again.

"How are you doing, Nicole?"

"Absolutely lovely."

"How do you feel?"

"Graceful and strong."

"Continue on."

The sky is azure, there are no puffy cumulus clouds to interrupt this bright blueness, and I am in my own world, high above everything. I want to do an arabesque on the log, but I think that will push Rachel over the edge, so instead I prance my way to the high end of the log. Once I'm there, Rachel has me stop and reflect again.

"How did you feel walking across that log with nothing to hold on to?" she asks.

"I felt strong and secure, and like I was suspended above the world. I felt serene."

"You have very good balance; I'm assuming this is from your years of gymnastics and ballet?"

"Yes."

Rachel had forgotten about my dance background. She likes to bring up that I have perfect posture, and that I don't have to be perfect. I wonder if she is advising me to slump, so I turn into an imperfect hunchback. I know that Rachel means no harm, and that she wants to help me get in touch with my emotions and mourn the loss and pain of my past. By breaking me down, she would be able to do that, but I won't let her. I can't let my guard down, and I can't let go. I have seen what happens when I am vulnerable, and I don't trust Rachel after my psychodrama.

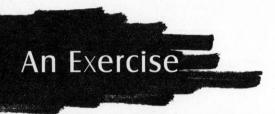

An Exercise

IN COMBATING MY PERFECTIONISM
AND SUPPOSED OCD

old therapist elaine that

I told Therapist Elaine that my graduate school GPA is a 4.0,
and she suspects that I have some perfectionist tendencies. Then
there is the vacuum cleaner incident. I am vacuuming Laura's side
of our room when her sheet gets stuck in the vacuum and starts a
minor fire. When I realize the vacuum cleaner is effectively broken,
I demand that I be allowed to borrow Second Floor's vacuum so I
can finish my side of the room. RC Evan challenges me to leave half
of my room unvacuumed as an exercise in challenging my obsessive-
compulsive disorder, which he diagnoses me with at that moment.

"I think you might have some OCD tendencies," says Evan,
suppressing a smile.

"I do not have fucking OCD, I'm just organized," I shout. "Why do you pathologize everything?"

I have been in treatment long enough to know that I am not going to get Second Floor's vacuum cleaner, no matter how much I beg, cry, or scream. I decide that if I am going to be treated like a mental patient, I might as well act like one, so I pitch a fit. I run down the hall screaming that all I want to do is vacuum my room, that Evan is a smug asshole, and that I most definitely do not have OCD; everyone knows odd numbers are disconcerting and everyone organizes the contents of their closet by color. All I want to do is vacuum my room. Evan asks me if I realize how immature I am acting, and I respond by throwing both my slippers at him. He pitches my slippers off the deck and onto the shore of the hospital lake that we have all dubbed Lake Bulimia because of the slimy, bright green algae blooms that cover the surface. Later, I sneak upstairs and smuggle the Second Floor vacuum to my room. This act solidifies Evan's belief that I have OCD, and he leaves Therapist Elaine a message about the vacuum cleaner incident.

Elaine concocts a therapy mega-assignment to address my negative body image, perfectionism, and OCD. Eliza is assigned the task of picking out a mismatched outfit for me to wear the next day, since this will help her conquer her passivity. I am to have no say in what I am wearing, and I have to wear the outfit all day.

Eliza comes to my room after dinner and searches through my closet and drawers, trying to put together a completely mismatched outfit. Because I don't wear much other than solid-colored shirts and jeans, Eliza has a hard time finding items that clash. Eventually she decides I am to wear my tan Guess tennis shoes, one black sock and one navy blue sock, my light blue paisley pajama pants with my knee-length jean skirt over them, and a black belt. I am also to wear a red long-sleeved shirt with a black tank top over it. I am fine until Eliza tells me I can't wear a bra.

I am to wear the outfit the entire next day, no matter how uncomfortable I am. I find relief in knowing that we are not scheduled to go on an outing—only the other residents will see me at my mismatched finest.

Then Recreational Therapist Douglas announces we are going to Barnes & Noble. I start crying and threaten not to go, so Laura says she will go mismatched as well so I won't feel quite so awkward. Laura wears a blue sundress with a long-sleeved black shirt underneath, and a pair of pajama pants. We roam Barnes & Noble together, two mismatched mental patients on an outing from the institution.

Revelations

nicole, you have an eating disorder.

"Nicole, you have an eating disorder."

"Oh my god, Holly, RC Julia says I have an eating disorder!"

"I'm just here for summer camp," says Holly.

We talk about making shirts with CAMP TURTLE POND FOR
THE NUTRITINALLY CHALLENGED printed on them, but we don't
get around to it.

Extended Metaphors

"This obstacle course symbolizes the road to recovery, with many pitfalls, wrong turns, and traps along the way," says Recreational Therapist Douglas.

"Your task is to direct your blindfolded partner through the obstacle course. If they step on a trap or make a wrong turn, they have encountered a setback or relapse. You can't help your partner unless they ask for help."

Holly blindfolds me and shouts out directions when I ask. I step on a few traps and relapse. Douglas tells me to "use my voice" and ask for help. I think this is a lame exercise, and I am tired of extended metaphors for recovery. After participating in my second extended-metaphor-for-recovery exercise, everything was drilled into my head. Use my voice. Ask for help. A relapse isn't the end of the world.

Douglas notices my bad attitude and asks if I want to talk about what is bothering me. I tell him no. No one in the group can understand why I hate extended-metaphor exercises so much. I think it's because I've been here too long.

Fortunately, Douglas gives us a break during our next Recreational Therapy and decides to drive us to Half-Price Books for an outing. The syllabus for my Reading Nonfiction: The Memoir class has just arrived in the mail. I pore over the list and decide I will buy as many of the books as possible at Half-Price Books so I can read them before school starts.

Armed with my list, I charge into the store, frantically looking for Sartre's *The Words*, Andre Aciman's *Out of Egypt*, Joan Didion's *Where I Was From*, and Paul Auster's *The Invention of Solitude*.

The store is disorganized, and all I can find is Paul Auster's *The Invention of Solitude* and Sartre's *The Words*. I track down RC Maria and ask her to help me look for books, but we can't find any more. How am I supposed to get my reading done? I am low on money since I haven't worked all summer, so I don't want to pay full cover price for these books, which I will have to do if I buy them from Barnes & Noble. I begin to panic. Everyone else in the class will have read the books. I will be behind. Everyone will think I am a lackluster and lazy student.

The other residents have bought psychology books (we are all trying to figure ourselves out) and murder mysteries. Holly buys books only if they have a pink and girlie cover. Laura has bought a slew of new serial-killer biographies that will be confiscated back at the EDC.

Everyone rolls their eyes at my purchases. They aren't surprised. I am one of the few residents who have not had to drop out of school because of their eating disorder. Therapist Elaine has posed the theory that school is my identity and that I am too wrapped up in it. I counter that it's healthier for school to be my identity than for me to identify myself purely as an eating-disordered person. I try to explain that I'm a graduate student and am passionate about writing, which makes me an eating-disordered scholar. Therapist Elaine says she understands that, but she thinks I take my perfectionism with school to the extreme. She is not the only person who has told me this, but I don't want to think about the consequences of her remark, so I banish it from my mind.

Sitting at the back table that evening, I am scrawling almost illegible scribbles in my journal while listening to Tori Amos's *Little Earthquakes*. I become aware of someone hovering over me, and when I look up, I see RC Evan mouthing something. I remove my headphones and hear him tell me to slow down, relax—I'm getting worked up. Step away from the pen and notebook.

"Look at how you're gripping your pen," he says. My fingers are clenched in an angry ball around my black-ink Bic (I write with black ink only; blue is too bright). "Why don't you come into the office and talk to me about what's going on?" says Evan. He doesn't understand that I can't talk about what is bothering me. I cannot verbalize the stream of ramblings that seemingly pour out of my pen and onto my journal pages. This is a purge substitute. I am purging the thoughts, memories, and voices that pollute my mind. I am purging the voice of my eating disorder, even if only temporarily.

The staff at the EDC feels that writing is my safe zone. They want to challenge me to express myself in different ways, such as painting, drawing, or other artistic forms. In high school, I loved painting class. I reveled in color and texture, but I could create only abstract paintings, or paintings that incorporated text. During Art Therapy at the EDC, I have the same problem, except I can't even do abstract paintings (staff says I can, just that my self-imposed standards are too high). Everyone challenges me to leave the realm of words and surrender to the realm of the abstract, but I cannot let go.

Prelude to Anger Management

july, and i'm angry It's July, and I'm angry all the time. I started this slow burn in
mid-June, after my parents flew to Wisconsin to visit, and now I am
up to fever pitch, slamming doors and scribbling furiously and illeg-
ibly in my journal. I have a bad attitude and take out my anger on
Recreational Therapist Douglas when he has us play a Twelve-Steps
game (I don't have a higher power, and this seems to be a problem).
When we do a symbolic extended-metaphor exercise in Psychodrama, I tell Rachel that I am sick of extended metaphors and that
they're stupid.

    Between dinner and evening snack, I lock myself in the confer-
ence room at the end of the hall because it's the most private place
on the floor. It has a glass door, so anyone can see in, but at least it's

soundproof and has a lock. I sit in the conference room and journal while listening to Dido if I want to calm down or Tori Amos if I'm feeling sorry for myself. If I'm feeling nostalgic and missing Pennsylvania, or just want to cry in general, I listen to the Tom Petty *Wildflowers* album and the tears drip off the end of my nose and smear the ink in my journal.

I need solitude to cry. I hate crying in front of the group, and I literally can't. But in the conference room I can sob as I journal, write letters, and finish my autobiography. Of course, someone inevitably checks up on me. Usually it is RC Julia. The other RCs, figuring that crying is therapeutic, leave me to my own devices. Julia knows better. Her shadow falls over the glass door, and I know she is there before she knocks. If I am crying, she will tell me I need to be around others and I need to get a snack (I usually attempt to hide in the conference room during evening snack time). I will protest that I'm not hungry and just want to be alone, but she will coax me out to the dayroom, where I'll curl up on a sofa with Eliza or Holly and snuffle, or fall asleep after eating a Cheerios bar.

The anger spirals into sadness.

Therapist Elaine wants to know about the anger, and I tell her I don't know why, I'm just angry all the time, at everything. She asks me to explore that "everything." When it is clear that my anger has reached a fever pitch, Elaine tells me we're going to try something different from traditional therapy. There will be no sitting on the sofa in the conference room, wrapped in my afghan. I am to come dressed for walking in the woods.

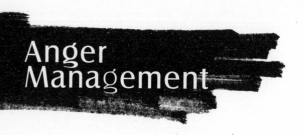

Anger Management

I meet Therapist Elaine in the RC office. She's wearing khakis, sandals, a long-sleeved shirt, and a jean jacket. I'm wearing capri pants, a T-shirt, and sandals. Elaine is holding a can of bug spray. I'm intrigued. We go downstairs to the kitchen, and Elaine requests a plastic bag filled with ice cubes. We walk out of the EDC and toward a path that leads to one of the lakes. This summer I have learned that Wisconsin has more lakes than Minnesota.

"I want you to think about everything that is making you angry, whether it is major or minor," says Elaine.

We trudge down the path and are assailed by a swarm of blood-hungry mosquitoes. Hard, white, itchy welts appear all over my feet, and I swat at the mosquitoes, but it does no good. Elaine lends me her jacket to cover my arms; even though it is eighty degrees, I wear it. There is something comforting about Elaine's jacket; I feel protected and safe in it.

Elaine and I coat ourselves in a sheen of bug spray while she tells me that I am to throw the ice cubes into the lake. Each time I throw a handful, I am to yell something I am angry about. I like this idea. My bag of ice cubes goes like this:

I am angry that I've gained weight.

I am angry that I'm spending my summer in treatment.

I am angry that I have no control over anything in my life.

I hate Dietitian Caroline because I'm gaining weight and she doesn't care.

I'm angry that I've wasted so much time thinking about calories, weight, and food.

I'm angry that I have heart problems at age twenty-three.

I hate my body.

I hate Minnesota.

I've used up my bag of ice, and Elaine is scavenging for rocks. I'm somewhat angry but am trying to avoid letting it build up, because I don't want to let go of the anger, because then I will break down and be sad. It is easier to be angry.

"Come on, Nicole, I've heard you scream—you can be much louder than this. I want to you to throw these rocks as hard as you can and scream about why you are so angry."

I'm angry that I am never good enough for my parents.

I'm angry that I'm not thin.

I'm angry that my parents won't let me tell my grandparents where I am.

I'm angry because I feel like I have no home.

"How are you feeling?"

"Somewhat irritated."

"You need to let go and be angry. I want you to scream it like you mean it and tell me the big things now."

I am shaking with emotion because I know I am not going to be able to fake this. There is no way out; it's just Elaine and me, the lake and the woods, and a pile of rocks representing my anger. I trust Elaine and I know this is my chance to let go; I have been waiting for and dreading this moment all summer. I am sweltering in Elaine's jacket and the mosquitoes are whining and buzzing around my head. I pick up a smooth, heavy rock and launch it into the lake.

I'm angry that Dirk is still teaching at Penn State Erie, and that I had to go through the ordeal of filing a sexual harassment complaint.

I'm angry that I carry this shame.

I'm angry that I'm not over this.

I'm angry that my uncle died.

I am furious and shaking. Elaine is searching for anything that I can throw into the lake. She sets a bunch of pinecones and sticks beside my feet.

She says, "You're getting louder and feeling more, but I know you can do better. I want you to scream over my voice. Come on,

Nicole, be louder, throw harder, scream, you can do better than that, louder, you have to be louder, scream . . . "

I'm angry that I keep everyone's secrets, I'm angry that I feel like this, I'm angry that I hate my body.

I feel strange, as if I am hovering above my body, watching this scene unfold from the trees. In technical terms I am dissociating, separating myself from my emotions because they are too intense and I am overloaded.

Elaine asks me to keep repeating what I am angry about as we walk back to the EDC, and I do. When we reach the EDC, I am completely inside my head, not very aware of my surroundings. I know there are residents outside and I am wearing Elaine's jacket and muttering about what I'm angry about, and I must look crazy with two large mosquito bites on my forehead.

Back inside, Elaine and I sit in the conference room and drink water because we are hoarse. Then she pulls out a hand mirror. She asks me what parts of my body I can tolerate or like. I say my eyes. I am to hold the mirror up to my eye and describe objectively what I see. I do this and we move on to my ear, then my elbow.

Elaine says we're done, and she asks me how I'm feeling. Her voice sounds distant, even though I know she's sitting across from me. I have an image in my head that keeps playing on repeat. I am thinking about Dirk's hands on my thighs as I lie drunk on his sofa, and then there is blackness and I keep wondering about the blank spaces in my memory. I can feel his hands on my thighs in the present moment. I tell Elaine this.

We walk down the hall to the RC office, where she has me sit across from RC Julia and hold an ice pack. I am to concentrate on the coldness of the ice pack and try to stay present. I clutch the ice pack and try to concentrate on the frozen pellets inside the plastic sheath. I read the instructions for use. But I can't block out the feelings of Dirk's hands on my thighs.

I am stranded in my memories, and time has stopped.

Faintly, I hear Julia.

"Nicole, it's Julia—you are in a safe place, no one is going to hurt you, and you are safe here. You are in Wisconsin, at the EDC; concentrate on the cold of your ice pack and keep your feet on the floor."

Someone touches me and I recoil. Julia is replacing my ice pack, since it's not cold anymore.

Gradually, I shift into reality. When I lift my head, I see Elaine and Julia. They have both been there the whole time. I am wearing Elaine's jacket and I don't know why, but it makes me feel safe.

"You had a flashback," says Elaine.

I feel shaky, weak, and drained. I give Elaine her jacket and spend the evening in the office with Julia, who talks to me about her upcoming wedding and her recent trip up north. She is keeping things light and keeping me distracted, and I am grateful. At one point in the evening, though, she breaks from her easygoing chatter.

"You must be so angry; I can't imagine how you feel right now."

"I hope you never have to find out."

Tornado Warnings

When I was younger, tornado warnings sent me running to the basement in a panic. Thunderstorms could induce major panic attacks in me within minutes, because they might produce tornadoes. As soon as I would see the warnings roll across the bottom of the television screen, I'd start to shake. One July day, back when I lived in Pennsylvania, I saw a funnel cloud descend from the sky in an off-white fury and skip gently across the hills on the other side of the river, just across from our property. I watched, entranced by the tornado's graceful beauty.

It is a summer of tornadoes in Wisconsin, and these are not the benign F1 twisters that Pennsylvania thunderstorms occasionally spawn—these are serious F3s that destroy houses and uproot ancient trees. I am at the EDC during the height of tornado season (May to August). There is no basement at the EDC, and that worries me.

One innocuous August evening, RC Julia clomps down the hall in her black boots, all business.

"We need to go down to Lower Level right now," she says.

"Why?" I ask.

"There's a tornado warning, and Lower Level is the safest place in the building."

My insides quiver as I gather my journal and the book I am reading. Holly and Laura are giving Julia a hard time. They think tornado warnings are a joke. They wouldn't think tornado warnings were so funny if they knew that the only way a person can survive an F5 is to ride out the twister in a bomb shelter–like structure.

The Lower Level hall is lined with eating-disordered patients of all ages and shapes. There are stick-thin teenagers text-messaging their friends on cell phones, there are obese middle-aged women knitting scarves in preparation for a Midwestern winter, and there are teenage boys with feeding tubes sliding out of their noses. Amid the residents are RCs in business casual, soothing the scared and nervous among us.

For once, I am not scared of the tornadic fury raging above me. Instead, I imagine the ecstasy of being swept into a funnel cloud, those few moments of rapture and flying, before almost certain death. I imagine being swept into the graceful, off-white funnel I saw in Pennsylvania, and how, I like to believe, I would simply surrender to the forces around me and not struggle.

WALKING GUIDELINES

1. **All residents must have a doctor's order to be eligible for walks.**
2. **Residents are to walk during scheduled times only.** Exceptions made for Wisconsin winter and summer weather. If a walk is missed due to cold weather, RCs can chose or not chose to do it later in the day if it warms up. Walks may not be done in place of programming.
3. The outside temperature must be 20° or above, with the wind-chill, in order for a resident to take any loops. If the temperature is above 85° the walk will be canceled. The RCs will determine if it is too cold or hot to take a walk. Walks should be done in the morning when it is cooler during the summer.
4. **Walks may be limited at the discretion of staff** due to (low vitals, pulse below 50, dizziness, noncompliance with meal plan etc.)

Excessive walking during a recreation outing may be deemed as your kind walks". Residents **may not** walk without staff if they do not have a doctor's order for "solo walks". Residents **may not** walk with other residents unless all of the residents have a doctor's order for "solo walks". "Solo Walks" **may only** be done during scheduled free time (not during programming). "Solo Walks" **may not** be done after meals. Residents that have solo walks, **may take** up to two "loops" and must remain on the walking path. Residents must remain on the hospital grounds for walks. Hickory Lane and the lake are off limits.

No walking after **6:00 p.m.** for **any residents.** Adolescents must always be walking with a staff member. "solo walks" and **may not** walk with other adult residents as their buddy. Adolescents **cannot** have Residents may only walk to the multi-purpose center and experiential "ropes course" if they are on "YELLOW" level or higher. Residents on ORANGE and RED must be driven to experiential by staff. Residents from one floor **may not** take walks with a resident from another floor. Residents that have "solo walks" need to take their walks during free time only and must notify their staff that they are leaving and need to sign out. Residents may lose the privilege of solo walks if they do not sign out or are seen abusing the privilege.

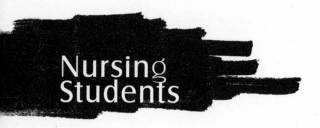

Nursing Students

Sarah and Michelle are nursing students from the University of Wisconsin–Milwaukee. They spend a month with us on the premise of learning about psychiatric nursing, particularly eating disorder patients. Sarah and Michelle arrive at the EDC in time to eat breakfast with us in the morning, and leave after our last group of the day.

They are fascinated and badger us with questions about our personal histories while we try to nap during free time. They volunteer to take us on walks around the hospital grounds and monitor us during snack time. At first we are on our best behavior around Sarah and Michelle, keeping our whining about weight gain and our disdain of Group Therapy to ourselves. However, as summer progresses and their psychiatric nursing rotation draws to a close, Sarah and Michelle see us at the height of our eating disorder–induced mania. They witness Danielle wail when she confronts a sofa cushion stained with crushed Oreos. They see Holly obsess for days about what flavor ice cream she will get for the snack challenge at Cold Stone Creamery. They watch bulimics tear down the hall after a meal or snack, fly into a bathroom, and purge before anyone can stop them.

It stings that Sarah and Michelle are our age. All of us are in our early twenties, and we are spending the summer in treatment because we have a nasty habit of sticking our fingers down our throats and horking up our food after a meal, or because we are so petrified of fat grams and calories that we abstain from eating most everything but the safest of foods (raw veggies, coffee, certain fruits). Meanwhile, Sarah and Michelle are in school, while many of us had to take a leave of absence or withdraw. They come dressed in professional attire, while we slink around the EDC in pajamas.

Sarah and Michelle are everything we are not. They are the type of women we could have been (and perhaps are) sans eating disorders. We begin to resent them—their delving into our pasts and case histories, their silent presence in Group Therapy, and their bright smiles.

At the end of one of my weekly individual therapy sessions, Therapist Elaine mentions that staff is concerned that I am becoming too close to Eliza, who happens to be a lesbian. I disclosed my bisexuality during Group Therapy shortly after my arrival at the

EDC, and was relieved when no one judged me for my sexual preferences. I assure Therapist Elaine that Eliza and I are just friends—we have a lot in common (we both live in the Twin Cities, we both are artsy nerds, we both purge), but we are not engaging in any romantic or sexual activity.

After individual therapy, I go to lunch with the rest of the floor and begin to think about what Therapist Elaine has implied. If I had been spending extra time with Sarah, a heterosexual resident, would staff have become concerned about our closeness? After lunch I inform Eliza about what Elaine brought up during our session, and we agree that we are being singled out because of our sexuality.

During the postlunch Group Therapy session, both Eliza and I speak about how we feel persecuted by staff because of our sexuality. Therapist Elaine is glad I am showing my emotions by yelling, which only angers me more. She is deflecting attention away from the issues at hand. All of the residents agree that staff is jumping to conclusions and acting in a ridiculous manner. I demand to know which staff member has informed Therapist Elaine of Eliza's and my troubling closeness, but she won't reveal who it was. I say that I wish that staff member had come to me personally instead of using Therapist Elaine as an intermediary.

Sarah and Michelle are outraged. They are convinced that staff is being homophobic. On our daily walk around the hospital grounds, Sarah and Michelle sputter with rage. Maybe it has something to do with their being our age and taking our side, but Eliza and I feel our anger and frustration are vindicated. For once, we are not the histrionic ones; we are not the ones jumping to conclusions and catastrophizing. Staff members are the ones who need to address their rigid beliefs, not us. We joke that staff needs a special Group Therapy session to address its faulty belief system.

I often wonder what Sarah and Michelle learned about psychiatric nursing while observing us. What memories of us did they take with them? Did they pity us? Did they think we were chronic, that we would never recover? Or did they see hope within us? Maybe they caught glimpses of our pre-EDC selves glimmering through the pale, vacant shells of our compromised bodies and starved minds. I wonder what they took from their experience at the EDC, those nurses-in-training.

Prank Calls

llo, this is dave from pizza hut

"Hello, this is Dave from Pizza Hut, and I have six large pizzas for delivery at the Eating Disorders Center."

"That has to be a mistake. This is an eating disorder treatment facility; no one here ordered pizzas," says RC Julia.

"Ma'am, I have to deliver these."

"You have to take them back; no one here is allowed to order pizza."

After Laura hangs up, we crack up. All of us were listening to the call, thanks to the speakerphone feature on my new cell phone. RC Julia really thought Pizza Hut was going to be delivering pizza. Later that night, Fred from Krispy Kreme calls.

"Hi, this is Fred from Krispy Kreme. I have an order for seven dozen Boston Creme doughnuts ready for pickup."

"I know this is a resident; you can stop now," says Julia.

Laura hangs up and we giggle.

It passes the time.

It's Fun to Weigh at the YMCA

After working out in the on-campus weight room for two weeks with Recreational Therapist Douglas, I graduate to working out at the local YMCA with a personal trainer, also named Douglas. My two afternoons a week of weight lifting with Recreational Therapist Douglas had consisted of ten minutes of jogging on the treadmill and light weight lifting. These sessions were frustrating, as I wanted to run longer and lift heavier weights; I wanted to burn calories and tone my body, which had grown flabby during my time at the EDC.

Recreational Therapist Douglas supervised everything I did in the weight room, but after my initial meeting with Personal Trainer

Douglas, I am turned loose in the YMCA for an hour and a half three times a week. Personal Trainer Douglas had worked with me on formulating a customized fitness plan that included small amounts of cardio and light weight lifting. I shelved the plan after our initial meeting, and instead headed to the pool, where none of the other EDC residents with YMCA privileges ever ventured, as the pool requires wearing a swimsuit.

Before entering the pool area, I go through the women's locker room, which is dangerous territory. In the locker room, I find the most secluded and dark corner and change into my swimsuit while glancing furtively around me, to make sure no one I know is in the locker room (several staff members belong to the YMCA). After I change, I stand in front of a full-length mirror and scrutinize my soft, pale body. Then I walk over to the scale, stare at it suspiciously, and step on gingerly, one hesitant foot at a time.

Even though I con Dietitian Caroline into disclosing my weight at least once a week, I cannot bypass the scale on my way to the pool. I have always been a scale junkie, sometimes weighing myself up to twenty times a day. During each of my short-term attempts at recovery, I threw out my scale, which meant that I then had to buy a new one when I succumbed to EDNOS. In the past five years, I've bought at least five scales.

After I weigh myself, I head out to the pool. The children's pool is adjacent to the lap pool, and I watch as the toddlers splash and giggle, slide down the slide, and generally have a good time. At the lap pool I jump in, wet my goggles, and secure my swim cap. In my pre–eating disorder life, I was a swimmer. Week after week at the YMCA, I struggle to find the rhythm I used to know as a girl on the swim team, the rhythm of steady breathing, even strokes, and a trim body that glides through the chlorinated water.

Instead, I splash and roll; I get water up my nose when I attempt a flip turn. I hate myself for being so out of shape; I hate my body for floundering in the water. Then, gradually, I develop a rhythm. I remember to breathe only on my left side, every third stroke, and everything slides together and I am swimming smooth, even strokes.

In the water, I am weightless.

At first, I can swim only three hundred yards. The next week, it's five hundred. The week after that, seven hundred. The EDC staff tells me I'm exercising too much. I tell them I just want to push myself. Secretly, I want to burn as many calories as possible. After my five-hundredth yard a voice invades my head, telling to me to go faster, swim harder. I'm not good enough. I'm not trying hard enough. It's the same voice that taunts me when I go running—it whispers, *Fat ass, fat ass.*

Despite my asthma, heart problems, and chronically low potassium, I listen to the voice. I swim until the last possible moment, sit in the hot tub for three minutes, weigh myself again to see if I lost weight during my workout, then catch the van back to the EDC, where I confess my transgressions to RC Marie and RC Allison. They relay what I tell them to Dietitian Caroline, who is not pleased and threatens to revoke my YMCA privileges if I find that going there is too triggering. I promise that I won't weigh myself, that I'll call the EDC if I need help. But I never do.

RC Marie tells me that she thinks about putting a note on the scale at the YMCA (she works out there in the morning, before her EDC shift) that says, Nicole, don't do it. Even though I know no one at the YMCA, the idea of RC Marie placing a note on the scale horrifies me. I beg her not to do it. And she doesn't, though part of me is touched that RC Marie cares enough to do something like that.

After I discharge from the EDC, I will avoid going to the gym. Then, to celebrate not having purged for six months, I will join the local YWCA. I will fall in love with the elliptical machine and the largest indoor track in the Twin Cities. I will go to the YWCA every day and spend up to three hours there, doing what I call cross-training: I will spend thirty minutes on the elliptical, run a mile, and swim hundreds of yards. This time, it won't be about calories and fat grams. It will be about realizing that my body, despite everything I have put it through, works fairly well.

The YWCA will have a digital scale that displays my weight to a tenth of a pound. I will hop on it before I go swimming and after I sit in the sauna, because maybe I have lost some water weight. I will begin to wonder how much my swimsuit weighs, and I will want to weigh myself naked, but I know people from school are members at the YWCA and I won't want them to see me naked. Curiosity will win in the end, and I will find out my swimsuit weighs less than a pound, and that I can sweat out up to half a pound of water weight in the sauna.

I will have transcendent experiences while listening to Liz Phair's self-titled album as I run laps on the track. All the anger, sadness, and rage will exit my body. This will be better than therapy. Perhaps my body has held on to all these emotions, and this is their only way out. I will begin to think sweating is a form of mourning. Our bodies remember.

The YWCA is where I will learn how other people live and move in their bodies. I will observe children running around barefoot in the Fit Kids Gym, I will watch mothers-to-be with rounded abdomens enjoying the sensation of weightlessness in the pool while they do prenatal water aerobics, and I will see a middle-aged woman with slashes across her chest from a double mastectomy sit naked in the sauna, unashamed. I will also bear witness to slender teenage girls stepping on the scale and berating themselves. I will want to tape a note to the scale that says, Don't do it.

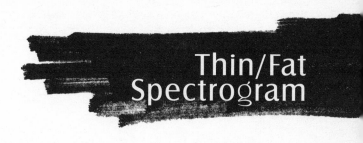

Thin/Fat Spectrogram

I rush, slightly sweaty, to the Psychodrama room after
working out under Douglas's watchful eye. Psychodrama Therapist Rachel is asking the residents how they feel today, and if there
is anything in particular they'd like to do a psychodrama about.
Everyone stares at the floor, and Rachel asks us all to stand up and
organize ourselves into a straight line from thinnest to not thinnest.
We stare at each other in horrified disbelief but do as we are told,
and all hell breaks loose.

Eliza and I know we are the two not-thinnest residents, so we
go to one end of the line, where we are challenged by Sandra and
Danielle, who try to shove us out of their way with their sticklike

arms. Both of them have a desperate gleam in their eyes. Laura places herself smack in the middle of the line. All of this happens in silence. Once we have arranged ourselves (for the most part) in a line, Rachel begins asking questions.

"Nicole and Eliza, how do you feel being the not thinnest in the group?"

"Strangely enough, I'm okay with it," I say, while secretly horrified.

"Yeah, I'm okay with it too," says Eliza.

Sandra and Danielle start shoving each other again.

"Sandra, do you really believe you are one of the not thinnest here?" asks Rachel.

"Yes. I should be at the front of the line."

"Nicole, do you think Sandra should be at the front of the line?"

"No. She's drastically underweight, while I am within my weight range."

"Can you see what Nicole is saying, Sandra?" asks Rachel.

"No."

This is the trouble with eating disorders: We all think we're the not-thinnest one in the room, and that we should be ashamed. Our distorted vision seldom lets us see the truth.

Body Image and Comparing

Sandra and Danielle are sitting on my bed while I search through my drawers for a shirt to wear. This is one of the days when I change clothes upward of ten times because nothing looks right. I walk to my closet in hopes of finding something there. Nothing. I stand in front of my closet in jeans and my bra, exasperated.

"You have a model-like torso," says Sandra.

"What?"

"Your breasts are the perfect size and you have a defined waist."

I realize that Sandra and Danielle have been evaluating my body, ranking my parts against their own. I grab a shirt from my closet, not caring that it doesn't fit like it used to. I don't want

Sandra and Danielle, neither of whom tops one hundred pounds, staring at my bare stomach anymore.

One day during Group Therapy, RC Allison hits on a source of my negative body image. I have just stated for the sixth time that day that I hate my body, hate looking in the mirror, and just want to hide in pajama pants and my Penn State sweatshirt for the rest of my life.

"Nicole, have you been comparing yourself to other residents?" asks RC Allison.

"Yes, every woman compares herself to others; it's not something anyone can help," I argue.

"I think you should try to remind yourself this is not an average group of women," says Allison.

She's right. I hate admitting that I am jealous of the anorexic girls, with knees they click together to hear the sound of bone hitting bone. I am jealous of how they have reduced their bodies to the bare essentials, how they are a lesson in symmetry and angles. My own body is all flesh and curves, thighs rubbing together, breasts bouncing, and hips that run into objects. Allison has sensed my misery. The anorexics stare at me with overly large eyes and the pinched faces of the starving.

Laura and Holly tell me that I'm beautiful, that I don't need to lose any weight. I suspect they are lying to me. It will take a long time for me to realize that the anorexic body is a symbol of sickness, and not something I should aspire to have. It will take even longer for me to learn to accept my own body for its unique planes and curves.

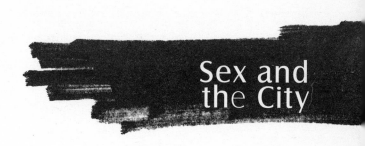

Sex and the City

hat are you doing up?

"What are you doing up? It's 4:00 AM."

"I have insomnia."

"I'm watching *Sex and the City* if you want to join me."

RC Shannon works third shift when Natalie is on vacation. No one wants to spend time with Natalie when they can't sleep, but I like Shannon, so I stumble down the hall to the dayroom, where I find her wrapped in a resident's blanket, watching *Sex and the City*. I curl up on the sofa and watch two episodes until I'm pleasantly drowsy, then head back to my room.

I savor the unit's quietness. No one is having a breakdown, refusing snack, having flashbacks, or screaming about weight gain.

It is August, three weeks before I discharge. I am sitting outside in a lawn chair, waiting for RC Julia to bring the van around for an outing. Everyone else is inside. The air is heavy with the scent of blooming flowers and the wetness of dew. The moment lasts until RC Marie pokes her head out the door and jokingly tells me to go back inside. I tell her how much I am enjoying the quiet, and she leaves me to enjoy it before the rest of the residents come out.

Julia Doing My Makeup

Danielle is knitting at the back table and no one is watching the Olympics, even though the television is blaring the results of the women's fifty-meter freestyle, when I come back from pass with $60 worth of Clinique makeup. I met up with Sandra at the Mayfair Mall, where she helped me pick out my very first eyeshadow duo, eyeliner, and undereye concealer stick.

My mother once told me that I could be a pretty girl if I just did something with my hair and started wearing makeup. So I cut off a foot of my hair and highlighted it, then bought some makeup because, secretly, I want to be a pretty girl.

RC Julia has promised that she will do my makeup for me

before I discharge from the EDC. There is a no-physical-contact rule at the EDC, which means staff is not supposed to touch the residents. Julia's offer to do my makeup violates that rule, so we both know she will have to do my makeover on a night when the floor is quiet.

Except for Danielle, all of the residents are napping. Julia agrees to do my makeup in the dayroom, before everyone wakes up. We take all of it out to the table where Danielle is knitting, and Julia paws through the various foundations, blushes, and lip glosses I now own while we talk about her recent camping trip. RC Julia is less than a year older than I am. I often wonder if we would have been friends if our paths had crossed outside of the EDC.

She starts with moisturizer, smoothing it onto my face in a circular motion. Next, she applies liquid foundation, and after that she brushes blush up my cheekbones. There is something soothing about the gentle, methodical way she applies my makeup. While she works on my eyes, I examine her face. I notice that her eyeliner is crooked and her eyes are a clear blue. Intimacy usually bothers me—normally I would feel exposed, sitting in front of Julia without any makeup. She can see all my flaws: my large pores, the black-heads that tend to dot the bridge of my nose, the patch of acne on my chin, my crooked front tooth, the fuzz on my upper lip. I do not think about any of this, though. I trust Julia. This kind and intimate gesture warms something within me.

Julia wants to apply my lipstick in the bathroom because the light is better there, so I perch on the counter while she concentrates on coloring my lips a rich plum. Afterward she turns me around to look in the mirror, and I want to cry. Who is this reflected woman with sultry green eyes and full lips? My impulse is to hug Julia, to thank her for making me feel so beautiful. But I don't. I remember the no-physical-contact rule and merely say thanks. We both stand in the bathroom for a minute, peering into the mirror.

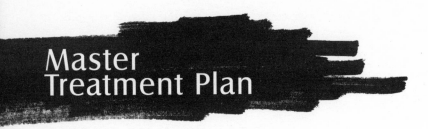

Master
Treatment Plan

8/13/04

DANGER/SAFETY ISSUES

High risk of relapse

Continues eating disorder behavior

UNMET GOALS

To remain abstinent from bingeing, purging, overexercising, and weighing self at YMCA

COMPLIANCE WITH TREATMENT

Patient is moderately compliant.

TENTATIVE DISCHARGE PLANS/DISPOSITION

Discharge 8/19/04. Resident plans to fly back to Pennsylvania and stay with a friend or in a hotel for a week and then drive back with a friend to Minnesota with her car. Treatment team for aftercare is being arranged. Resident is continuing to decide if she wants to begin school right away, or take a semester off. If she takes a semester off, resident plans to find a full-time job.

Therapeutic Exercise:

GETTING READY TO LET GO

When is enough enough? I don't know. The health problems, the lost time, and the loss of myself should be enough, but it's not. I've made progress, I've talked, I've been working on my issues, but I haven't let go. I don't know how to let go of so many things in my life, including the eating disorder. I don't know why I'm not living my life to the fullest. Maybe I don't know how.

Something is missing, but I don't know what. Maybe it's that I feel I don't deserve to live life to the fullest, whatever that means. I don't think it's that I'm scared. Sometimes I don't think I'm a very good person. I feel guilty, and I hate myself. I feel like I deserve this eating disorder and the pain it brings with it. My eating disorder and school go hand in hand. I'm scared to go back to school without my eating disorder, because I'm afraid I won't be such a good student without it. I like the physical release of purging. I don't know how to deal with feelings, and I don't want to deal with feelings. I don't know what it will take for me to let go. If I knew, I wouldn't be here. I'm not ready to let go.

Part of me is ready to let go, but the other part isn't. I want to want to let go.

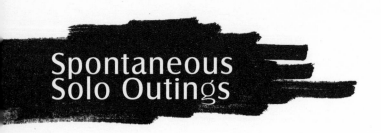

Spontaneous
Solo Outings

first i don't understand why

At first I don't understand why everyone wants to sneak out to their car and drive to the gas station for coffee when staff is busy. I find this behavior immature and adolescent. Then, after my second month of limited opportunities to have caffeine and unsupervised time, I begin to understand.

Sandra and I stay behind during a Barnes & Noble outing so that we can sneak out. We are supposed to be working on discharge planning. Sandra sneaks out to her station wagon, and I pretend to go on my solo walk around the hospital grounds. I jump into her station wagon and duck until we are off hospital property.

The back seat of Sandra's car is filled with candy wrappers and half-filled bottles of Diet Coke, and a peculiar odor is wafting through the air. I think back to a Group Therapy session when Sandra confessed that she binged and purged in her car, discarding half-eaten food, wrappers, and containers filled with vomit in the back seat. I begin to breathe through my mouth and I pull my legs up to my chest, rather than placing my feet on the floor.

Sandra drives slowly, not paying attention to the road. A minivan almost collides with us at an intersection. I yell at Sandra to speed up—we have to be back before anyone notices we are gone—but she keeps dawdling and talking about how green the fields are in Wisconsin.

At the gas station, I make a beeline for a twenty-ounce bottle of Diet Code Red Mountain Dew because I crave the manic anxiety that caffeine induces. Sandra samples different flavors of coffee and experiments with flavored creamers. I yell at her to hurry up. Back at the EDC, I slip in and no one notices, even though I am so hyper I can barely sit through Group Therapy.

That night, Elise and I head to the gas station. Instead of sneaking out, we make a dash for her car, sprinting across the lawn, which is slippery from the torrential downpour of a recent thunderstorm. Elise screeches out of the parking lot and swerves onto the road. Her driving is the opposite of Sandra's: She speeds down the wet roads, going sixty when the speed limit is thirty, pulling out in front of cars, and making left turns on red.

I have never felt so free in my life.

Instinctively, I know Elise is a reckless driver and my life is probably in danger, but I believe I am in charge of myself, and the wind is cool and fresh on my face and I feel alive.

A Surreal
Moment

It is ten o'clock on a Thursday night in August, less than a week before I discharge, and I am sitting in the office with RC Erica and RC Marie. My new obsession is the game Scattergories. Therapist Elaine challenges me to play it a few times, to see if I can play without getting too competitive (her suggestion stems from a half-court volleyball game during which I knocked RC Allison over in my attempt to spike the ball). I want to play Scattergories all the time, and RC Marie jokes that it's all I talk about. Erica and Marie finish their charting early and are up for a game or two. Then Elise comes in and wants to play after she hooks up her feeding tube, and so does Danielle.

Sandra comes back from pass loaded with bags of clothes she shoplifted from the mall; she will confess her thievery later that night. She also wants to play. All six of us sit in the office; the residents are on the floor in their pajamas, and Erica and Marie sit at the computer desks. We talk and laugh, and I think I'm content for the first time in a long time. Earlier in the evening, RC Marie told me that she could see my personality emerging as my eating disorder receded. She told me it was so good to hear me laugh, and to see me smile genuinely. I will miss RC Marie, and her stories about working at Planned Parenthood and the trials of raising two small children.

The feeding pumps are making a rhythmic, soothing noise; Marie is singing some song about all the states in the nation that no one is really listening to; Sandra is waving her arms triumphantly; and RC Erica is trying to give Elise her evening meds. I am laughing at the ridiculousness around me.

I want to pinch myself to see if I've dreamed the last three months.

Therapeutic Exercise:

THREE STAGES OF RECOVERY

RECOVERY: I'm living my life fully and not focusing on or distracting myself with eating disorder behaviors. I own my life and recovery. I'm attending my outpatient appointments and actively striving for recovery. I'm enjoying my life and realizing that each new day is a fresh start. I'm using my support system and not isolating myself. I am honest with myself and others. I am not engaging in eating disorder activities, but if I slip, I realize I can move on. I am following my meal plan and expressing my feelings. I will take time out for myself every day and combat my perfectionist tendencies. I will remember to breathe and take care of myself, and remember how far I've come.

IN-BETWEEN: Some days I am more recovery-oriented than others, but I will stay focused and ask for help on hard days. I will realize recovery is not an overnight process. The following behaviors are indicative of this stage: weighing myself, skipping appointments, not talking, purging sporadically, skipping meals, overexercising, bingeing, losing weight, feeling overwhelmed and out of control. I will seek out extra support and talk more. I won't keep secrets, I will reexamine the motives for my behaviors, I will challenge my thinking, and I will journal. I will also seek further treatment if appropriate. I will realize this is a hard time, and I will not give up on myself.

RELAPSE: I have relapsed, but I will keep working, asking for help, and believing in myself. I will seek more intensive treatment. These behaviors indicate relapse: purging every day, weighing myself multiple times a day, taking diet pills, abusing caffeine, fasting, restricting, overexercising, isolating, dropping below my weight range, fainting, worsening health problems from not taking care of myself, feeling like there is no way out, and going through the motions of my life. If I find myself in full relapse, I will be honest with my treatment team and support system. I will consider a higher level of care. I will get labs drawn regularly. I will talk and not keep everything inside. I will accept and evaluate how I ended up in a relapse.

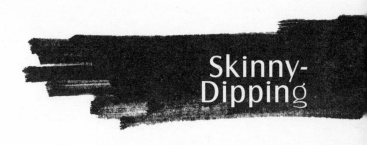

Skinny-Dipping

lly has never skinny-dipped before

Holly has never skinny-dipped before, so we decide to meet up on pass and search the numerous local lakes for a secluded spot where we can forgo swimsuits. Residents are strictly forbidden to meet up with each other on pass, but Holly and I never heed that rule. I leave my rental car in the Stone Creek Coffee Shop parking lot, and she picks me up. Most of the time, we drive to a suburb of Milwaukee and get large Caramel Coolers at Caribou Coffee. Sometimes we drive into Milwaukee and get coffee at Alterra, a coffee shop near the shore of Lake Michigan.

We also eat meals together while on pass, which is perhaps the biggest rule that we break. Often when residents meet up with each other on pass, it is for the purpose of bingeing and purging together. Holly and I never do that. We talk each other into eating and out of purging after a filling meal. When we both discharge and move back to the Twin Cities, Holly will invite me over for dinner and invite me out to eat when I am in the midst of restricting and relapsing. I will sit with her after eating and distract her from purging, and I will talk her out of stopping at Perkins and bingeing.

On the last Saturday before Holly discharges, we meet up as usual. We drive with the windows of her Mazda down as we drink quarts of Diet Coke and listen to the Dixie Chicks on the stereo. Our plan is to drive the isolated country roads around the hospital and search for the perfect spot to skinny-dip. We have not anticipated finding the numerous private property and no trespassing signs we encounter. We decide to alter our plan and head to Lake Labelle, a local lake with a beach and docks.

We have to stop at Kwik Trip for more contraband Diet Coke and to change into our swimsuits. The two of us squeeze into the tiny bathroom, turn away from each other, and undress. Holly wears her favorite blue and green one-piece, and I wear my black and green two-piece. It goes against reason that I feel comfortable in my swimsuit, with my stomach and legs exposed, but I do. I feel that my body is proportional, and that I have nothing to be ashamed of. Besides, other than the hospital residents and staff, I know no one here.

I have a picture from that day, taken by an anonymous sun-bather. Holly and I have shed our towels and are facing the water.

Our arms are around each other's waists and we appear apprehensive yet happy. When I get the film developed, Holly and I agree it is a flattering picture of both of us. It proves we are not the obese, cellulite-riddled women we think we are. I keep returning to the picture; it marks the beginning of acceptance for me—acceptance of my body, acceptance of myself—and the ability to finally just let go, even if only for a short while.

We are tentatively hopeful on the day we go skinny-dipping. Holly has been in treatment for eight months, I for two and a half. We are learning to let go and accept ourselves, but what no one has told us is that the hardest part lies ahead, after treatment. Both of us will struggle and relapse. I will restrict and lose all the weight I gained at the EDC and then some. I will land back in the ER, dehydrated, orthostatic, and with a slow, erratic heartbeat. Holly will begin purging again, return to treatment, and end up on a feeding tube. But we don't know this yet. We are convinced that we are almost there, that we have almost beaten our eating disorders.

The water is cold from this rainy summer in southeast Wisconsin, but we swim out to the anchored rafts and clamber up the slick ladder. We lie side by side on the raft and sunbathe while talking intermittently about the other residents, staff, and our families back home. Holly is from a suburb of St. Paul, and she has been trying to convince me to return to the University of Minnesota in the fall so that we can go to school together.

The sunlight gives my pale skin a light brown hue. I've spent most of my summer inside the over-air-conditioned EDC, so I don't take this day at the lake for granted; I savor the warmth of the sunlight streaming over my skin. I will be sunburned, but I don't care. For one afternoon I am a normal twenty-three-year-old sunbathing with a friend, not an eating-disordered patient rating my body image on a scale of one to ten.

"Ready to jump back in? I'm getting hot," says Holly.

"Yeah, let's do it," I say.

The coldness of the water shocks my warm skin and I bob to the surface, teeth chattering.

"We're far from shore; no one will notice if we take off our suits," I say.

"Okay. Can you imagine what Therapist Elaine and Dietitian Caroline would say if they knew we met up on pass and skinny-dipped?"

"They wouldn't know whether to congratulate us for doing something positive to improve our body image or yell at us for meeting up on pass," I say.

Holly begins the process of peeling off her bathing suit while I work on the strings on the top part of my two-piece. Eventually I give up and pull the top over my head, then slip off my bottoms easily.

Our bodies are pale white, tinged with green from the water. We tread water and swim around, careful not to lose our grip on our suits.

"This feels really freeing," says Holly.

"I told you it feels good."

We manage to slip back into our suits and swim to shore. When we are done swimming, we drive to Milwaukee for coffee, then split up. If we arrive back at the EDC at the same time, it will appear suspicious. So we stagger our returns, thinking no one will be the wiser. However, we are both sunburned and have Lake Labelle admission bracelets on. Staff figures it out.

Therapist Elaine is annoyed, but Dietitian Caroline is proud of us for challenging our body-image issues, although she doesn't condone skinny-dipping at a public beach. A few weeks later, the whole floor decides to go to Lake Labelle on an outing, but it isn't the same. Sandra immediately starts swimming laps in an attempt to burn off the beef enchiladas she ate for dinner, Laura has a rape flashback, and the anorexics are in the water for only five minutes because their lack of body fat makes them more sensitive to the cold. RC Julia sits on the shore, dressed in long pants and a long-sleeved shirt on a blistering, eighty-five-degree day. It is apparent that we are from the EDC.

Sandra, Holly, and I remove our swimsuits, but I am self-conscious now, as Sandra is thinner than I am. The outing goes further downhill when Holly jumps off the anchored raft and yells, "I'm a raging bulimic." RC Julia isn't amused, and she threatens to cancel the rest of the outing, which includes going to Cold Stone Creamery for a snack challenge.

At Cold Stone I order a small Birthday Cake Remix, the same thing I get every time we go there. I sit outside with RC Julia, Holly, and Sandra, who keeps eating my ice cream. As I scoop the sugary ice cream into my mouth, I contemplate how my thighs touch at the top, how my upper arms are really too large these days, and how I think I saw a double chin when I looked in the mirror this morning.

I could tell RC Julia that I'm struggling with urges. I could sit down in the office after we get back from Cold Stone and stay there until the urges pass. I could journal and break down the thoughts behind the urges. But I don't. Instead, I deconstruct my body, part by part, flaw by flaw. And when we get back to the EDC, I sneak down the hall when no one is looking. Above the toilet is a list of reasons why I shouldn't purge. I read over them, stick my finger down my throat, and heave until nothing but stomach acid comes up. No one hears me do this. I've perfected the art of the quiet purge.

Afterward, I pace. I am jittery and red-eyed. Finally, I confess to RC Julia that I purged. She asks me why I didn't come find her or someone else and talk about my urges. I want to tell her that the voice in my head, the voice of bulimia, is too loud and that there are no alternatives. I want to tell her how scared I am that I will never recover, that I will spend my life in a constant state of anxiety about calories, fat grams, exercise, and purging. But I don't. I tell her I don't know. And she tells me to keep fighting.

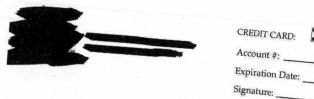

CREDIT CARD: **VISA**   MasterCard

Account #: _____

Expiration Date: _____

Signature: _____

Amount to be Charged: $_____

JOHNS NICOLE

8/19/04	JOHNS NICOLE			
	BALANCE FORWARD	1009722		
9/30/04	PAYMENT	24,500.00		
	*** TOTAL DUE ***		9,000.00-	15,500.00
				15,500.00

_____ At this time, your co-pay amount is: _____
__✓__ Insurance has been billed on your behalf. This is only a statement for your records.
Any questions, please call ██████████ or ██████████
   For Inpatient stays – Ext. ███
   For Residential Eating Disorder and Chemical Dependency – ██████████
   For Residential OCD, Child & Adolescent Center and Partial Hospital – E██████████

DISCHARGE SUMMARY

		UNIT: EDI	**ROOM:** -
PATIENT NAME:	JOHNS NICOLE	**MEDICAL RECORD #:**	
ADMIT DATE:	05-24-2004	**DATE OF BIRTH:**	06-29-1981
DISCH. DATE:	08-19-2004	**SEX:**	F
ATTD. PHYSICIAN:			

CHIEF COMPLAINT:

HISTORY OF PRESENT ILLNESS:

<u>ADMISSION WEIGHT</u>: 133 pounds.

<u>DISCHARGE WEIGHT</u>: 140 pounds.

COURSE IN PROGRAM: The patient was admitted and initially did quite well in terms of her eating disorder symptoms although struggling with a lot of difficulty with food, weight and concerns in terms of body image, which was quite significant for this patient. She also struggled with a past trauma history, issues around relationships with parents and feeling a great deal of ambivalence in terms of those relationships, more than anything a great deal of difficulty kind of dealing with uncomfortable emotions and talking openly and honest about how she feels without reverting to eating disorder symptoms. The patient was able to work a great deal on improved outlook, improved self-esteem, improved problem solving and also improved body image which, although was somewhat of a struggle during her treatment she was able to really make significant strives.

She did attend the YMCA on a regular basis, struggled initially with a lot of difficulty around compulsive weighing, however was able to significantly abstain from this type of behavior and again made pretty significant improvement in terms of those symptoms.

We did talk at length about potential benefit of either an SSRI for what appeared to be some ongoing anxi symptoms of possibly the use of Topamax in terms of ongoing binge urges however, Nicole was not interested in these options and I felt that this was reasonable. However I did encourage her to consider th as options in the future if she were to struggle after discharge.

LABORATORY STUDIES ON ADMISSION: Notable for potassium on 08-09 3.6, on 08-05 3.8. Chemist panel and blood count only notable for abnormal potassium of 3.3 on 08-04. Potassium 3.7 on 08-02, 3. 07-29. Normal chemistry panel and blood count on 07-26. Normal phosphorous, magnesium and potas on 06-21. TSH low of 0.02 on 06-01. Free T_3 within normal rage Free T_4 1.24, potassium 3.5 on 06-07. chemistry panel notable for TSH of 0.07 on 0 Potassium 3.8 on 06-10, 4.0 Negative urine drug screen.

in terms of her eating dis...
concerns in terms of body image...
trauma history, issues around...
of those relationships, more than...
ns and talking openly and honestly...
tient was able to work a great...
also improved body image...
was able to re... make significant...

problem...
tment sh...

s... ...ced initially with a lot of difficulty around compulsive
...abs... from this type of behavior and again made pretty
...symptoms, ... was reasonable, however I did encourage her to consider these
...t potential benefits of either an SSRI for what appeared to be some ongoing anxiety
...ssibly the use of Topamax in terms of ongoing binge urges however, Nicole was not
...these options and I felt that th... was reasonable, however I did encourage her to consider these
...in the future if she were to struggle after discharge.

LABORATORY STUDIES ON ADMISSION: Notable for potassium on 08-09 3.6, on 08-05 3.8. Chemistry
...el and blood count only notable for abnormal potassium of 3.3 on 08-04. Potassium 3.7 on 08-02, 3.4 on
07-29. Normal chemistry panel and blood count on 07-26. Normal phosphorous, magnesium and potassium
on 06-21. TSH low of 0.02 on 06-01. Free T$_4$ 1.24, potassium 3.5 on 06-07. Free T$_3$ within normal rage of
4.0. Negative urine drug screen. Potassium 3.8 on 06-10, chemistry panel notable for TSH of 0.07on 05-25
and potassium 3.3.

DISCHARGE MEDICATIONS: (1) Zyrtec 10 mg daily. (2) Prevacid 20 mg daily. (3) Potassium chloride 20
mEq p.o. b.i.d.

DISCHARGE PLANS AND RECOMMENDATIONS: The patient was discharged medically and
psychiatrically stable. No suicidal, assultive, or homicidal thoughts, behaviors or impulses. She was going to
followup in Minnesota (St. Paul/Minneapolis) area.

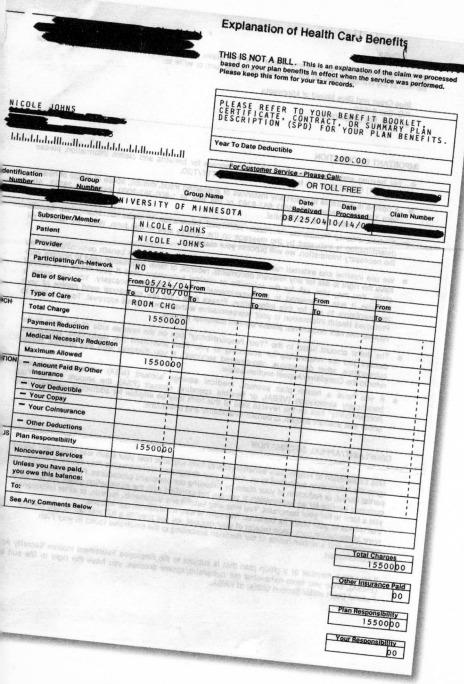

Explanation of Health Care Benefits

THIS IS NOT A BILL. This is an explanation of the claim we processed based on your plan benefits in effect when the service was performed. Please keep this form for your tax records.

NICOLE JOHNS

PLEASE REFER TO YOUR BENEFIT BOOKLET, CERTIFICATE, CONTRACT, OR SUMMARY PLAN DESCRIPTION (SPD) FOR YOUR PLAN BENEFITS.

Year To Date Deductible   200.00

For Customer Service - Please Call: OR TOLL FREE

			Group Name					
Identification Number		Group Number	UNIVERSITY OF MINNESOTA		Date Received 08/25/04	Date Processed 10/14/0	Claim Number	
Subscriber/Member			NICOLE JOHNS					
Patient			NICOLE JOHNS					
Provider								
Participating/In-Network			NO					
Date of Service			From 05/24/04 To 00/00/00	From To	From To	From To	From To	From To
Type of Care			ROOM CHG					
Total Charge			1550000					
Payment Reduction								
Medical Necessity Reduction								
Maximum Allowed								
− Amount Paid By Other Insurance			1550000					
− Your Deductible								
− Your Copay								
− Your Coinsurance								
− Other Deductions								
Plan Responsibility								
Noncovered Services			1550000					
Unless you have paid, you owe this balance:								
To:								
See Any Comments Below								

Total Charges	1550000
Other Insurance Paid	00
Plan Responsibility	1550000
Your Responsibility	00

Purge

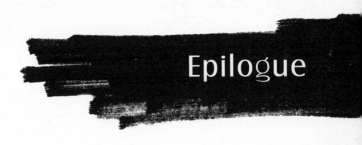

Epilogue

And now: it is easy to forget
what I came for
among so many who have always
lived here . . .
—FROM "DIVING INTO THE WRECK," BY ADRIENNE RICH

Holly abandoned me for the safety of bulimia the October
after our summer at the EDC, but we began to drift apart long
before then. It started after Holly discharged but while I was still
at the EDC, living in the parallel world of treatment—back before
those nights of drinking martinis at her house in the suburbs,
before the revelry of homecoming weekend, before the very first
day of school.

"It was a slip," she says.

I lie stretched out on the EDC sofa in my pajamas, wrapped
in my ivory afghan, contemplating what to say. In the RC office, RC
Caroline is dispensing evening meds and telling the residents a story

about her two-year-old son. Residents are sprawled on the day-room furniture, watching television, knitting, and talking on their cell phones. The EDC environment is safe; we are protected from ourselves while we are here. Holly is in the real world, where no one checks up on you 24/7 and no one pulls your head out of the toilet.

"Were you honest with your treatment team?" I ask.

"Yes."

Holly has been in and out of treatment since she was fourteen. Some professionals consider her a chronic case. She has been to the EDC two times already, and she will go back again less than six months after her "slip."

"A slip is just a slip; it's not a relapse," I say.

"I know. I'm not going to let this mess me up."

At first Holly does well; she doesn't let the incident affect her recovery. Then she is hospitalized with a gastric motility disorder caused by her bulimia, which means her stomach does not digest food the way it's supposed to. Instead, food sits in her stomach long after it should have been digested, and causes acid reflux and nausea. Holly has bout after bout of uncontrollable vomiting, which triggers her dormant bulimia.

After Holly is discharged from the hospital, she begins purging. At first she tells me not to worry about it, it's no big deal, she's not doing it that often, but I see where this is headed. However, I can't say much about Holly's relapse without being a hypocrite, as my own motivation for recovery is dwindling. While I'm not purging, I'm just not eating. The urge to restrict is insidious. I cut back my meal plan a little bit at a time, until I've lost fifteen pounds and end up dehydrated, with low electrolytes, hooked up to a heart monitor in the emergency room. Any time I question Holly's purging, she questions my lack of consumption.

I manage to turn my relapse around, and by spring semester I'm eating enough to function and have started exercising. Then Holly goes back to the EDC in late January, and I'm left to fend for myself. Without Holly, I have no one who understands my struggle; I have no one to call when I need help. My non-eating-disordered friends grow frustrated and tell me I have to eat—I simply have to eat.

One night in December, before Holly leaves for the EDC for her third round of treatment, I call her from Rainbow Foods on East Lake Street. I have been wandering around the grocery store, searching for something to eat for dinner. Every time I lift an item from the shelf, I glance at its caloric content and place it back on the shelf. Nothing is safe enough for me to eat, as I am in restriction mode. I call Holly in desperation; I need someone to tell me what to eat, and that it is okay to eat.

"I've been wandering around Rainbow for the last hour, and I need you to tell me what to eat," I say.

"How about a Lean Cuisine?" Holly says.

"That's too much food," I say.

"Actually, that's similar to your meal plan."

"I can't do it. Please just tell me it's okay to eat microwavable soup."

"Nicole, it's perfectly fine to eat microwavable soup."

"Thanks. I'll call you after I eat."

Because Holly has given me permission to eat, I rationalize that it must be okay. I am too ashamed to call my non-eating-disordered friends and ask them for help, and if I called my therapist every time I had an eating disorder quandary or crisis, I would be on the phone three-quarters of the day.

Every day post-treatment presents a new challenge in my recovery from EDNOS. There are the bakeries I pass on my drive to school, there are the catered lunches for the Introduction to Creative Writing teaching assistants, there is the problem of eating a snack during the break in seminar, and then there is my ever-rising anxiety and panic before seminar, which I stifle by swallowing Xanax tablets with Diet Coke in a bathroom stall before seminar begins.

Holly understands all of this.

And then she leaves—she goes back to the safety of bulimia, then back to the safety of the EDC, with its regimentation and therapeutic schedule, and I am left to fend for myself in a world in which I have forgotten how to live.

At the EDC, there are no doors to lock. You don't have to remember to take the trash out on Tuesdays, to turn your head-lights off, to pay the phone bill or do your homework. When I first left the EDC, I forgot to do those things and the world closed in on me in a screaming frenzy of demands. Less than two weeks after discharging from the EDC, I am back in Minneapolis, teaching, taking classes, and trying to readjust to the world. There was no transition time for me; unlike Holly, I did not have the opportunity to participate in a partial hospitalization program or an intensive outpatient program. I went from 24/7 therapy to one hour of therapy per week.

In retrospect, why I relapsed in the fall is no mystery.

My therapist wanted to send me back to treatment, but I refused. I was afraid I'd become a lifer, one of those women who are constantly caught in the revolving door of treatment.

I can understand how Holly relapsed. I understand how, even though she had damaged her body irreparably, she kept engaging in bulimia. My understanding scares me. Other people don't understand. And I don't want to anymore.

In January, when I begin spring semester, Holly begins the EDC program for the third time. We talk on the phone every night, but something is different. I don't find Holly's evasion of the EDC rules hilarious anymore. All I can see is that she is hurting herself by sneaking in contraband, going on spontaneous solo outings, and harassing staff.

Holly tells me that the staff members always ask about me. I am in the habit of writing them letters about school and how I'm doing; she tells me they love my letters and are so proud of me for recovering. I imagine that the fact that I am succeeding and she is failing grates on her. There is an awkwardness between us.

In February I win a fellowship to the Prague Summer Program, and that convinces me to recover fully. I am going to Prague and I'm going to enjoy it. I am not going to spend a month there with my head over the toilet, or passing out on cobblestone streets because I haven't been eating.

At the end of the month, I drive to Wisconsin and visit Holly. The EDC staff is happy to see that I am happy, healthy, and whole. Holly is sporting a nasogastric tube when I visit, a testament to the fact that she is not happy, healthy, and whole.

We go to the mall, we go to Milwaukee, and we sit in the dayroom and talk (which is a bit trippy, since I'm an ex-resident). I cry when I leave.

Holly calls me a few weeks later and tells me she wants to die, and I don't know what to say. I think about how many friends I've taken to the emergency room since college, how many of them wanted to die, and how I never know what to say in the face of all that pain, because anything said in that moment sounds trite. All I can do is listen to her ragged breathing and sobs and tell her it will be okay.

In May, when I drive home to Pennsylvania, Holly is still at the EDC, so I stop in Wisconsin to visit her. Staff tells me I should come back to the EDC as a motivational speaker because I'm doing so well. I tell them I can't do that while Holly is there; it would be a big slap in the face. Holly and I say goodbye for the summer.

I call her from Prague. She sounds so happy to hear my voice, and while I'm excited to talk to her, I'm not as excited as I thought I'd be. In Prague, I've remembered how to live. I haven't weighed myself for a month, I haven't counted calories, and I haven't declared any foods off-limits. For the first time in a long time, I am genuinely happy. I take only one Xanax the whole month.

In August, when I return to Minnesota, Holly is hospitalized in the Mayo Clinic because she can't keep any food down, even if she wants to. She gets a nasojejunal feeding tube.[1] She gets sicker in September. She spends the whole month of October in the hospital after a failed surgery. Now she has two tubes, one in her stomach and one in her jejunum. I drive down to the Mayo Clinic and find Holly high on pain medication, a shell of herself.

When Holly returns home, I visit her. We watch *America's Next Top Model*. Cans of feeding-tube formula sit on her kitchen counter, along with a suction device that attaches to the tube jutting out of her stomach. Dark circles ring her eyes, and walking is a struggle. One day, I spend the afternoon with Holly while her parents go to work. They don't have any more vacation days left. We spend the day watching television and napping. Holly sobs as she packs her surgery wound with sterile gauze. After she has injected narcotic pain medication into her tube, I lie beside her on the bed until she falls into a drugged sleep.

On Halloween, Holly's dad calls to tell me that she has to have emergency surgery to clean out an infection that her feeding tubes have caused in her abdomen, and that her surgeon has warned her family that she might not live. After I hang up the phone, I start sobbing uncontrollably. I drive to a local park and sit among the leaves, crying because I am so scared I could lose Holly.

Holly is septic, and when the surgeons open her abdomen, they remove a liter of pus. For the next three weeks, she clings to life in the ICU. I visit her every day.

The first day is the hardest. At the hospital reception desk, I am asked if I am a relative or a friend, and I lie and say I'm her sister. I ride the elevator up to the ICU and think about everything that has happened since I met Holly. I think back to that summer day at Lake Labelle when we skinny-dipped, and about how much things have changed for both of us over the course of a year.

Holly's parents, sisters, and grandparents are all crammed into her ICU room. Her dad shouts in an overly excited voice, "Hey, Holly! Nicole's here!" I set my bag on the floor and walk gingerly over to her hospital bed. Holly is hooked up to more tubes than I can count, and she has the light blue pallor of the dying. Her pupils are dilated and her hair is plastered to her forehead in a sweaty tangle. I am scared to touch her.

"Nicole, I knew you would come," she says.

She drifts back into unconsciousness, and I hold her bloated hand. Her mom tells me that Holly is on three different IV antibiotics to try to kill her infection, and that her organs are failing. Her heart beats an arhythmic thirty beats per minute, her oxygen levels are low, her kidneys are shutting down, and she's alternating between high fevers and abnormally low temperatures. Her brain swells and she has massive seizures. Her prognosis is not good.

The worst day is when Holly is almost comatose, and has her head thrown back and mouth open, with the feeding tube hanging out her nose. She looks like Terry Schiavo.

For the next three weeks, I jump whenever my phone rings, scared that it might be Holly's parents calling to tell me she's died. I cry in my car when I listen to the Dixie Chicks and all the songs we used to listen to at the EDC. I develop a routine: I go to school, then go to the ICU afterward. I grade creative writing projects while sitting with Holly, occasionally holding her hand, giving her sips of water, and telling her where she is when she startles awake.

At night, the ICU is blanketed in silence save for the soft whir of the machines attached to Holly and the soft tread of the nurse's rubber-soled shoes. When I try to grade writing projects, my gaze wanders out the window, where the Cathedral of St. Paul is lit bright against the murky glow of the urban night sky, and I wonder if Holly will ever wake up to see this view. At night, in the ICU, when I'm driving home and when I'm in class, my mind drifts back to summer at the EDC, and I wonder how Holly and I ended up where we are.

---

1. A nasojejunal feeding tube goes through the nose into the small intestine (jejunum) and bypasses the stomach. These types of tubes are used for people with stomach motility problems.

Acknowledgments

many people have helped me

So many people have helped me both recover and write this book. I'd like to thank all of the staff at the treatment center for giving me the tools to enter recovery, and for their extensive support. Salina Renninger, PhD, and Nicole Grunzke, PsyD, for believing in me and helping me see that recovery was something I could attain. My colleagues and professors in the University of Minnesota MFA program, especially Julie Schumacher, thesis adviser extraordinaire and BFF. I'd like to thank my student groupies for their relentless encouragement and faith as well as the fine people at the Mercersburg Academy who nurtured my love of reading and writing, and the members of the English department at Penn State Erie, who taught me about the writing life and encouraged me to pursue an MFA. Liz, for your friendship and love through all of this. Agent Barbara, for being the most amazing agent a writer could ever wish for, and Brooke Warner at Seal Press for her enthusiasm and dedication to *Purge*.

I would also like to thank the Prague Summer Program for the generous Eda Kriseova Nonfiction Fellowship during the summer of 2005 as well as the Vermont Studio Center for an Artist's Grant that allowed me to finish *Purge*.

Most of all I'd like to thank Brady Johnson, the love of my life and best friend.

About the Author

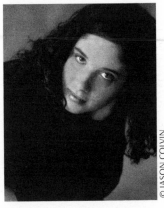

© JASON COLVIN

Nicole Johns was born and raised in rural western Pennsylvania and has a BA in English from Penn State Erie and an MFA from the University of Minnesota. She resides in Minneapolis with her soon-to-be husband, Brady Johnson, and has been in recovery from her eating disorder since 2005.